ADHD

workbook for adults

Myths and Facts, Tips and Tools to Improve Concentration, Overcome Work Challenges, Improve relationships, Love Yourself, Take Charge of Your Life and Break Through Barriers.

RACHEL FREEMAN

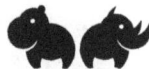

IPPOCERONTE
publishing

~ CONTENTS ~

~ Chapter 2 ~
# TREATMENT OF ADHD

~ Chapter 3 ~
# OVERCOMING ADHD PROBLEMS IN REAL LIFE

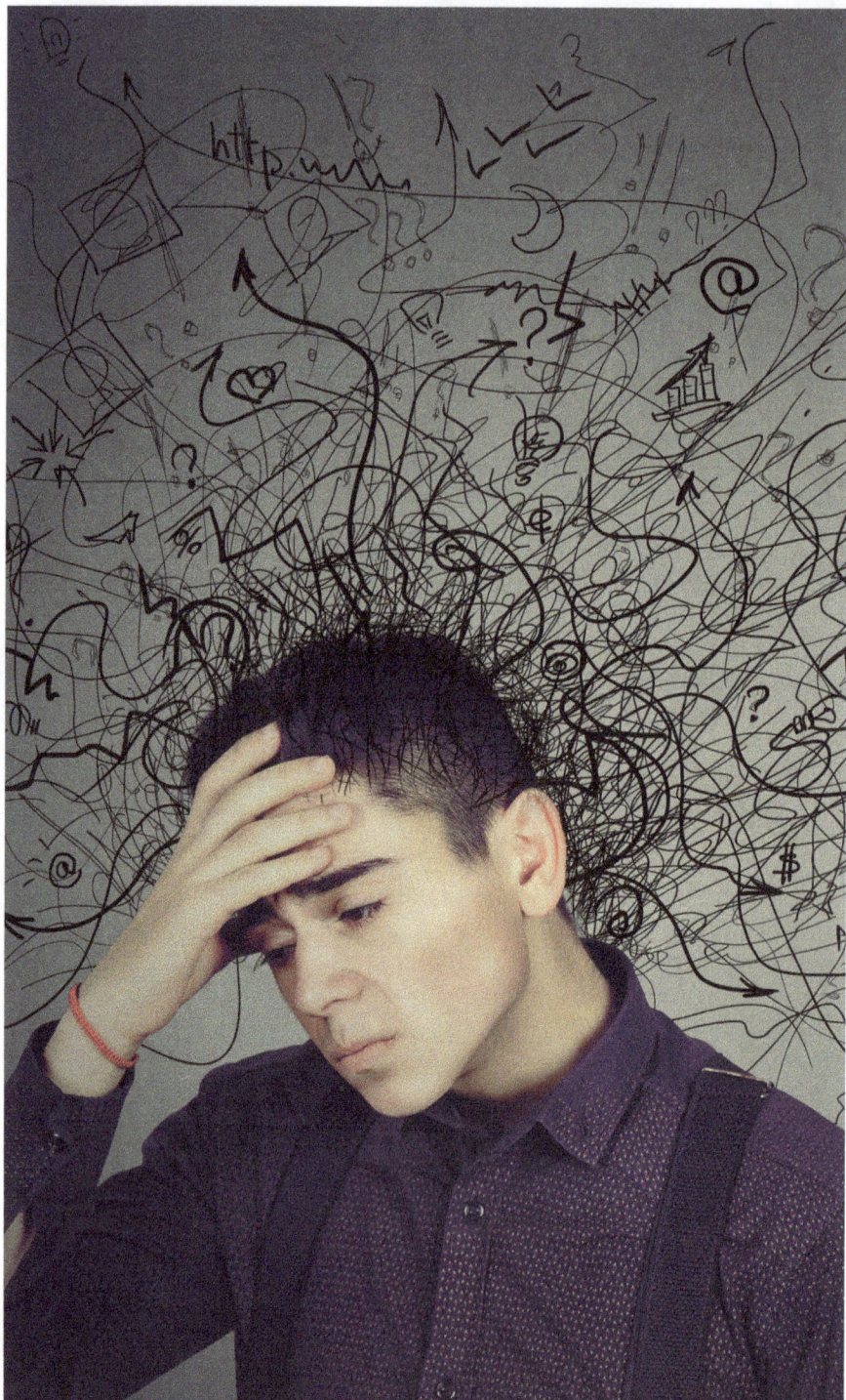

~ INTRODUCTION ~

ADHD used to be known as a childhood disorder, but it has achieved widespread recognition as a problem for adults, too. However, people do not develop ADHD in adulthood. It starts as a childhood disorder and progresses into adulthood. According to research, over 60 percent of children who develop ADHD do not outgrow or correct it ("Grow Out of ADHD? Not Likely," 2020).

The disorder eventually continues into adulthood, greatly affecting the quality of one's life. However, some people with ADHD do not receive a diagnosis in childhood. The disorder goes unnoticed, and this often poses a problem during diagnosis.

Adults with ADHD start to suspect problems when they trace the history of their academic struggles and frequent job changes (or outright inability to keep one). Most of them have more problems in their personal lives than others of similar circumstances. Many of them cannot keep relationships, including friendships, and may get into more trouble with the law. Many have frequent traffic violations and have no trouble dropping out of school.

It is possible for people with ADHD to live a normal life despite being undiagnosed, but they usually put in extra effort than an average person to get through important life milestones. Many of those diagnosed in adulthood believe life would have been better if the diagnosis had come earlier. ADHD is known to be more common in males than females, hence the erroneous belief that it only occurs in males.

ADHD can be treated with medications and therapy. There are other practices that can help provide relief from the symptoms. Adults with ADHD are often at a loss on how to manage their condition and seek all the help and support they can get.

This book intends to be a valuable addition to the resources available for people with ADHD. The author studied psychology and is a life coach working with ADHD patients and had a personal encounter with a close family member diagnosed with the condition. This book is a way to contribute to the support of people with ADHD. In this book, you'll find useful information on ways to combat ADHD and improve your quality of life.

CHAPTER 1

ADHD: AN OVERVIEW

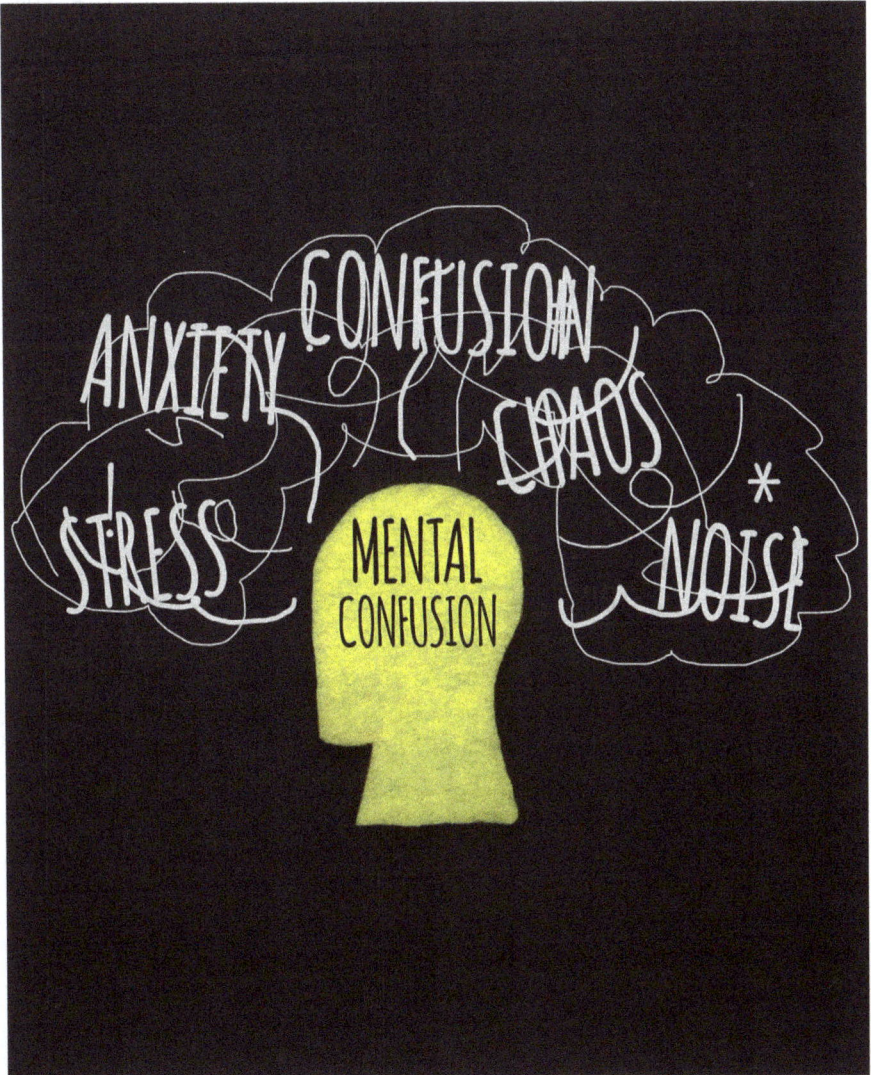

WHAT IS ADHD?

ADHD is a condition that affects the development of the nervous system, including the brain. This condition often develops in childhood at around seven years old, although close monitoring might notice it before this age. Children who have this disorder have difficulty with hyperactivity, impulsivity, inattentiveness, distractions, and task completion.

Although ADHD poses a huge concern for parents and guardians, the condition is easily treated. Following the onset of ADHD symptoms in childhood, many cases often progress into adulthood. Adults with the condition have a heightened form of the symptoms which began in childhood. They regularly struggle with remembering information, focusing on and managing tasks, or following directions.

The symptoms of this disorder that progress from childhood to adulthood without care or management may cause developmental problems for the individual. An adult with this condition might lead a poor quality of life because of problems affecting their academic, social, behavioral, emotional, and vocational skills.

ADHD presents in three forms:
1. Inattentive Presentation
2. Hyperactive Presentation
3. Combined Presentation (A combination of hyperactive and inattentive behaviors)

All three forms of the condition are the developmental functions that are most affected. In cases where the symptoms are unclear, the child is said to have "Unspecified ADHD." Until recent times, the inattentive presentation was thought to be a different condition. Now, it is properly categorized as a major symptom of ADHD. Attention Deficit Hyperactive Disorder affects around 11 percent of children aged four to seventeen (Legg, 2018). The onset of symptoms occurs around age three to six, although the condition is mostly detected and diagnosed at the average age of seven. When left untreated, the condition persists into adulthood. In America, 4 percent of adults above eighteen struggle with several symptoms of ADHD (Legg, 2018).

In a society where people quickly classify various ailments as mental illnesses, it is important to understand that ADHD is a neurodevelopmental illness. While mental illnesses affect people's moods, thoughts, and actions, ADHD is a behavioral disorder. It simply means the individual does things differently and doesn't mean something is wrong with them. Classifying this disorder as a neurodevelopmental disorder is more accurate because it affects the neural pathways in brain performance, causing behavioral problems at different developmental stages.

In disassociating ADHD from mental illnesses, it should also not be categorized as a form of autism or even a learning disability. ADHD and autism are neurodevelopmental disorders. They exist independently and express different symptoms, and many children who have autism display symptoms of ADHD.

This disorder is not a learning disability, even though the symptoms may pose a learning challenge. Like autism, many children with Attention Deficit Hyperactive Disorder can have a learning disability.

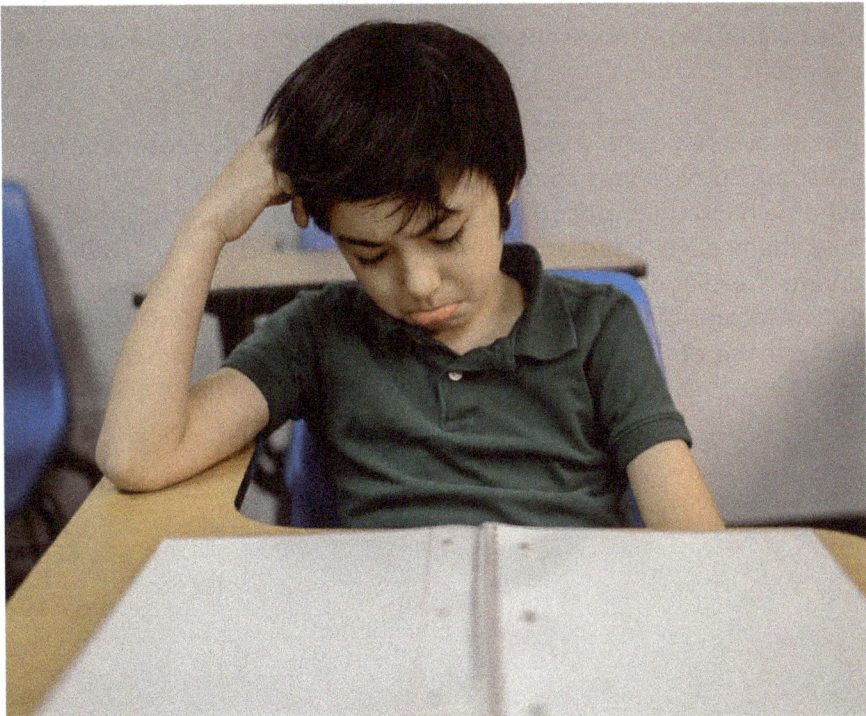

ADHD IN ADULTS

ADHD symptoms lessen as a child ages. Still, some adults experience major symptoms that prevent them from having a high quality of life. Most adults with this disorder have no idea that they have it, especially if there was no diagnosis during childhood. These adults just know that they have trouble meeting up with everyday tasks.

Attention Deficit Hyperactive Disorder may become noticeable when the individual is a child or an adolescent. It is possible that as children, they were scolded for their symptoms. The most common form of ADHD in adults is the inattentive form. This is usually because as children grow with the disorder, they tend to drop the hyperactivity and restlessness, but still have trouble with concentration and risk taking. As a result, they have a harder time interacting with others.

It is not uncommon for people with this disorder to have anxiety, depression, abuse drugs, or fail to cope in less structured environments. It could also be because children who have the inattentive form of ADHD go undiagnosed since they are not hyperactive (which is easily observable). So, no one notices that they have this disorder until they are adults.

This usually happens in women and girls. They could present as more quiet and timid even among peers who do not have ADHD. They eventually go on to become adults and may not get a diagnosis until they themselves have a child who is diagnosed with ADHD. Only during the diagnosis of their children will they come to understand the symptoms of the disorder and how similar their behavior patterns are to those of their child and begin the journey to get help.

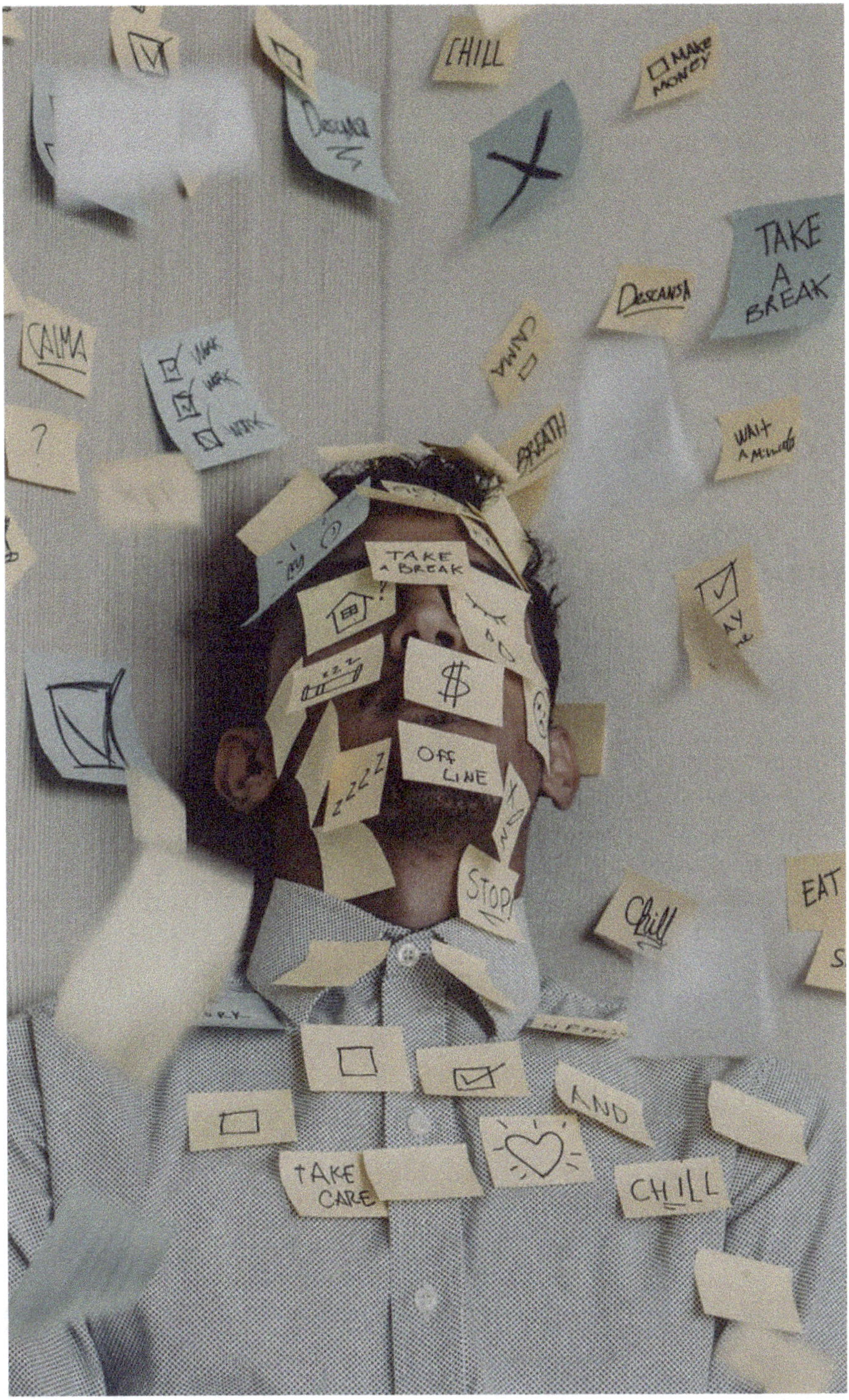
CHILL
MAKE MONEY
TAKE A BREAK
DESCANSA
CALMA
TAKE A BREAK
OFF LINE
STOP!
Chill
EAT
AND
TAKE CARE
CHILL

SYMPTOMS OF ADHD

If you think you have ADHD, you might want to cross check your symptoms. Generally, adults with Attention Deficit Hyperactive Disorder have difficulty with

- concentration
- recollection
- organization
- punctuality
- following rules

The symptoms can either be mild or severe and can create problems in different spheres of their life.

CHALLENGES ADULTS WITH ADHD FACE

These are some problems an adult with ADHD may have:

- anxiety
- chronic boredom
- chronic lateness and difficulty remembering things
- depression
- anger issues
- lack of focus when reading
- work problems
- impulsiveness
- mood swings
- trouble sustaining relationships
- lack of motivation
- bad organization skills
- low self-esteem
- low frustration tolerance
- substance addiction

If these adults are students, they may have trouble with their academic performance, repeating grades, following rules, and may drop out of school.

If they have jobs, they'll typically record poor performances and change jobs frequently. They are prone to getting a speeding ticket, license suspension, or being involved in car crashes. People with ADHD are almost always in financial peril. They may experience marital issues and are, in many cases, separated from their spouses or divorced.

TYPES OF ADHD

ADHD, as touched upon earlier, exists in three forms.

The Hyperactive and Impulsive Type

Individuals with this form of ADHD get the urge to be on the move constantly. It is difficult for them to stay calm and seated. When they are children, they seem to be fuelled with strange amounts of energy and run around a lot. Both children and adults with this type are talkative, interrupt others, and lack self control. This type of ADHD is very common among men and children.

For a person with Attention Deficit Hyperactive Disorder to be classified under the Hyperactive-Impulsive type, they must have up to six out of nine of the following symptoms:

- standing up often when seated
- squirming
- fidgeting
- interrupting others
- being talkative
- constantly moving with high energy bursts
- trouble playing quietly
- constant blurting out
- talking out of turn

Inattentive Type

Individuals with this type of ADHD usually make easily avoidable mistakes, and have trouble keeping to concise instructions or arranging tasks and activities. The reason for their inattention is usually due to poor working memory and they misplace items a lot. This type is most common among adults and girls. Long ago, it was known as ADD. For a person with ADHD to be classified under Inattentive type, they must have up to six of the following seven symptoms:

- missing important details
- ignoring conversations
- lackadaisical
- not willing to follow or understand instructions
- losing important things needed to finish projects
- dodging tasks that require hard work
- regularly distracted

Combined Type

This type of ADHD is very common. Individuals with Combined type ADHD have symptoms of the Inattentive type as well as those of Hyperactivity and Impulsivity. For a person to be classified under the Combined type ADHD, they must have six or more symptoms of Hyperactivity and Impulsivity and six or more symptoms of Inattention.

CAUSES OF ADHD

Attention Deficit Hyperactive Disorder is a neurobiological disorder with symptoms that are partially dependent on the environment of the child. There are different causal factors of this disorder which scientists have identified, listed down below.

Heredity

ADHD can be caused by genes and runs in families. Parents who have the disorder can pass it on to their children. A child can also have Attention Deficit Hyperactive Disorder if other family members have it. However, this does not imply that every parent with the disorder will by default pass it to their child. A child is 50 percent more likely to have ADHD if one parent has it (Bhargava, 2021). There is also a 30 percent chance of having it if a sibling has it (Bhargava, 2021).

Based on estimations, over 70 percent of people with the disorder have the disorder as a result of genetics (Collingwood, 2016). Still, children can inherit genes without activating them. While the genes are necessary to cause the disorder, there has to be interaction between several of them, as well as the environment, before the symptoms can manifest. When children inherit ADHD from their parents, they are not bound to have the same type of ADHD as that parent. ADHD is also not a sex linked gene, and can be inherited from either a mother or a father.

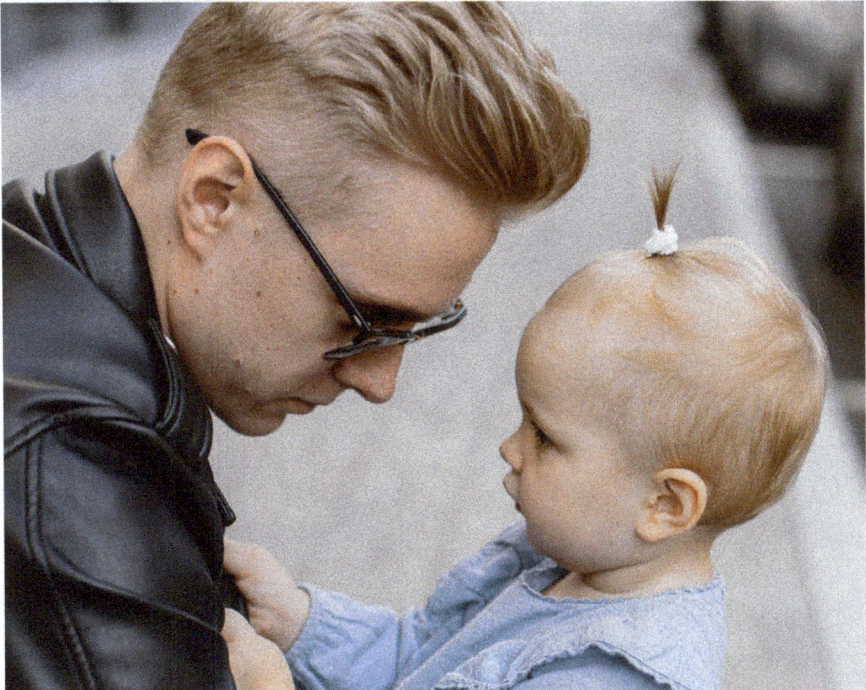

Problems During Pregnancy

The circumstances of a mother during pregnancy can contribute to her child getting diagnosed with ADHD. Premature births, low birth weight, and difficult pregnancies all contribute to the risk of having ADHD. From research, babies born to women who smoked or drank alcohol during pregnancy have higher chances of developing ADHD (Weinstock, 2017). Being exposed to lead, PCBs, and pesticides during pregnancy may also be a factor.

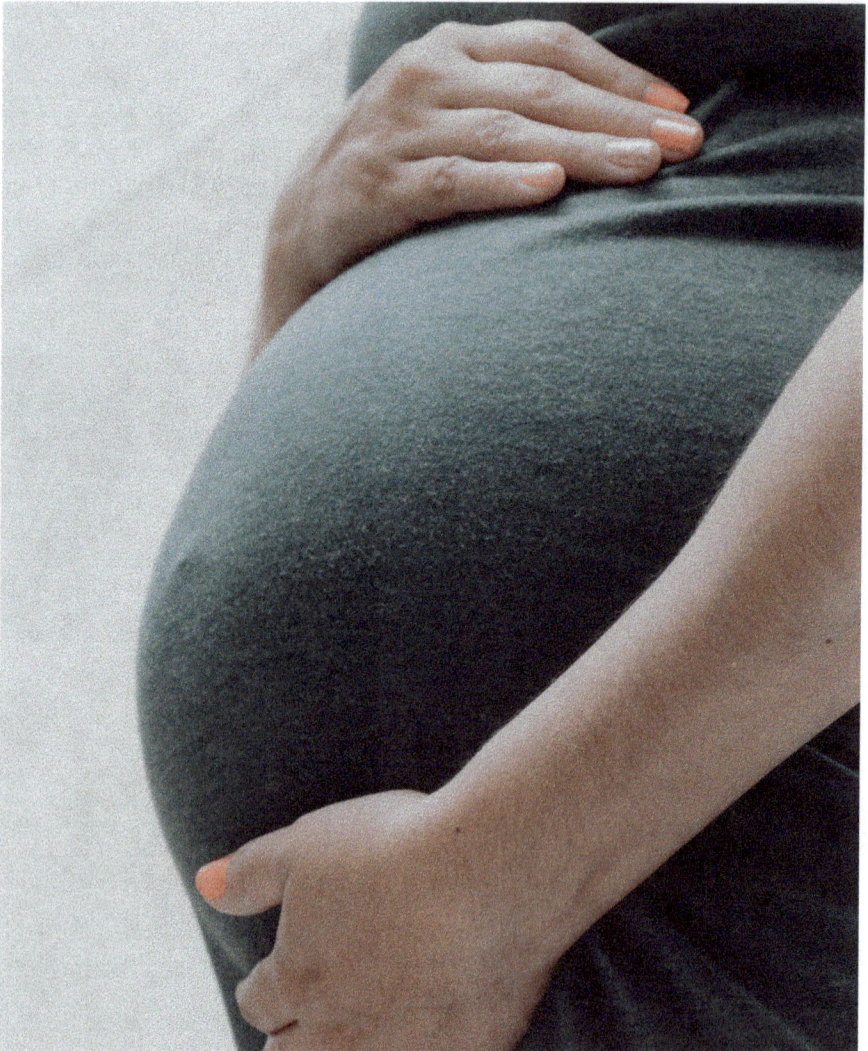

Toxins

Toxins in the environment are harmful to pregnant women and infants. On rare occasions, these toxins can cause ADHD. Exposing a child to high quantities of lead or other toxins leads to an interference in brain development, which eventually affects behavior and other development.

Brain Anatomy and Function

Attention Deficit Hyperactive Disorder is often linked to a reduced level of activity in the brain, specifically in the parts responsible for controlling attention and activity level. Children who are exposed to head injuries affecting the frontal lobe of the brain, the center for emotion and impulses, often develop ADHD. Oftentimes, ADHD is caused by major head injuries.

Because there are no exact causes of ADHD, people tend to blame the onset of the disorder on several other factors. ADHD is not caused by any of the following:

- food additives
- high sugar consumption
- parenting styles
- poverty
- stress
- playing video games
- immunization
- diet or allergies

DIAGNOSIS OF ADHD

If you have suspicions of this disorder, you need to know what is involved in the diagnosis.

Diagnosing ADHD in Children and Teenagers

A child can only be diagnosed with ADHD if they have up to or more than six symptoms of either Inattentiveness type or Hyperactivity and Impulsiveness type. In addition to the above criteria, they need to have

1. Started displaying symptoms before 12 years old.
2. Had detectable symptoms for a minimum of six consecutive months.
3. Showed symptoms in a minimum of two different settings. For instance, displaying symptoms at school and at home to erase the chances that the attitude is simply the child's reaction to teachers or parenting methods.
4. Showed symptoms that cause them to have a harder academic, social, or occupational life.
5. Showed symptoms that have no link to developmental disorders or difficult phases, and cannot be explained by other conditions.

Diagnosing ADHD in Adults

Getting an ADHD diagnosis as an adult is quite difficult due to conflicts on the relevance of the symptoms used for children and teenagers. Sometimes, an adult is diagnosed if they meet up to five or more of the symptoms of the two types of ADHD listed in diagnosing children.

Usually, the symptoms presented by the adult must have an interference in their work or education, driving skills, and friendships and relationships. The problems or symptoms must not have developed recently in adulthood for it to be considered.

While there is no single genetic, medical, or physical test for adults with ADHD, qualified mental health care professionals can provide diagnostic evaluation by collating information from various sources. Here are some sources.

ADHD SYMPTOM CHECKLISTS

They include

- A concise history of past and current behaviors.
- Standardized behavior rating scales.
- Information gotten from different family members or acquaintances who are very familiar with the individual.

Some professionals include tests of cognitive ability and academic achievement as a way of ruling out learning disabilities. For adults, the diagnosis doesn't come simply from a discussion with the individual or a short observation during office visits.

This is obviously because the person's symptoms may not be displayed during office visits and the physician can only diagnose when there is accurate knowledge of the person's history. The physician also has to consider the chances of having co-occurring conditions.

The diagnosis of ADHD for adults is based on clinical guidelines from the fifth edition of the diagnostic manual, Diagnostic and Statistical Manual of Mental Disorders, or 'DSM-5', obtained from the American Psychiatric Association.

The guidelines from the manual are applied both in research and clinical practice. The evaluation process will determine how regular the symptoms manifest and if they have been present from childhood.

INTERNET SELF-RATING SCALES

It's not uncommon to find individuals diagnosing themselves of several conditions following internet research. Most people use questionnaires and symptoms lists from some internet sites to confirm if they have ADHD or not. However, there are no scientific validations for these questionnaires and so people need not use them.

The only valid diagnosis for this disorder should come from a qualified, licensed professional. Even if you suspect that you may have the symptoms and you pull out several questionnaires to support that suspicion, it remains invalid unless confirmed by a professional.

QUALIFICATIONS NEEDED TO DIAGNOSE ADHD

The importance of getting a diagnosis for ADHD from a qualified and licensed mental health professional cannot be overemphasized. Professionals that can give a diagnosis include clinical psychologists, physicians (family doctor, psychiatrist, neurologist, as well as other types of physicians), or clinical social workers.

Confirm from the professional how much training and experience they've had in treating adults with ADHD. The expertise and knowledge a professional has about ADHD is often more relevant than the qualifications or degree they have. Many qualified and experienced professionals provide information about their knowledge and experience with patients. Professionals who are unwilling to share this information may not be the right choice for you.

FINDING A QUALIFIED PROFESSIONAL

One of the easiest ways to find a qualified health practitioner competent in ADHD care is to get a referral from your personal physician or GP. Another good option is to reach out for recommendations from a local university-based hospital, a medical school, or a graduate school in psychology. It will also help to lookout for ADHD support groups around you and discuss it with those who attend the group.

It is highly possible for most of them to have used the services of professionals in the area. Get them to link you with qualified ones. If your insurance has cover for this treatment, you can check for professionals in their list. They can also help you find a healthcare professional. Alternatively, you can look online for lists of providers of ADHD, like CHADD'S professional directory and others.

If you think you have any of the signs of ADHD, you need to get checked with a qualified health professional and desist from self-diagnosis.

PREPARING FOR AN ADHD EVALUATION

The idea of an ADHD evaluation can be overwhelming for some people. At times, people feel nervous and have feelings of being abnormal. Being nervous is normal, but there is no need to fear an ADHD evaluation. If you suspect that your major life issues might be related to ADHD, then do well to seek help without judging yourself. Usually, people misconstrue ADHD as a problem for only children and the idea of an adult having it seems like a reason to avoid responsibilities.

ADHD health professionals find it necessary to review their patient's old school records. Bring the records to your first appointment if you have them. Remember to present reports of any past psychological testing. If your symptoms affect your workplace, you should also present any job evaluations done to your doctor.

The professional you choose might need you to fill out questionnaires before evaluation, and also indicate which of your closest relations will act in some parts of the evaluation.

HAVING A COMPREHENSIVE ADHD EVALUATION

While the ADHD testing procedures and materials differ from one health care professional to another, there are certain standards needed to be met in a comprehensive evaluation. A comprehensive evaluation must have a detailed diagnostic interview, unbiased statement from a spouse or close family members, DSM-5 symptom checklists, and standardized behavior rating scales for ADHD, including other psychometric testing introduced by the professional.

ADHD DIAGNOSTIC INTERVIEW

The ADHD diagnostic interview is the most vital part of a comprehensive ADHD evaluation. It requires the detailed history of the person and can either be structured or semi-structured. In the interview, the person is made to answer some predetermined, standard questions to boost reliability and prevent the possibility of varying conclusions from different interviewers.

The health professional talks about many different, important topics, and asks follow-up questions to ensure full coverage of all areas of interest. The health care professional will also crosscheck the diagnostic criteria for ADHD, noting which of them applies to the person both at the time of the interview and since childhood.

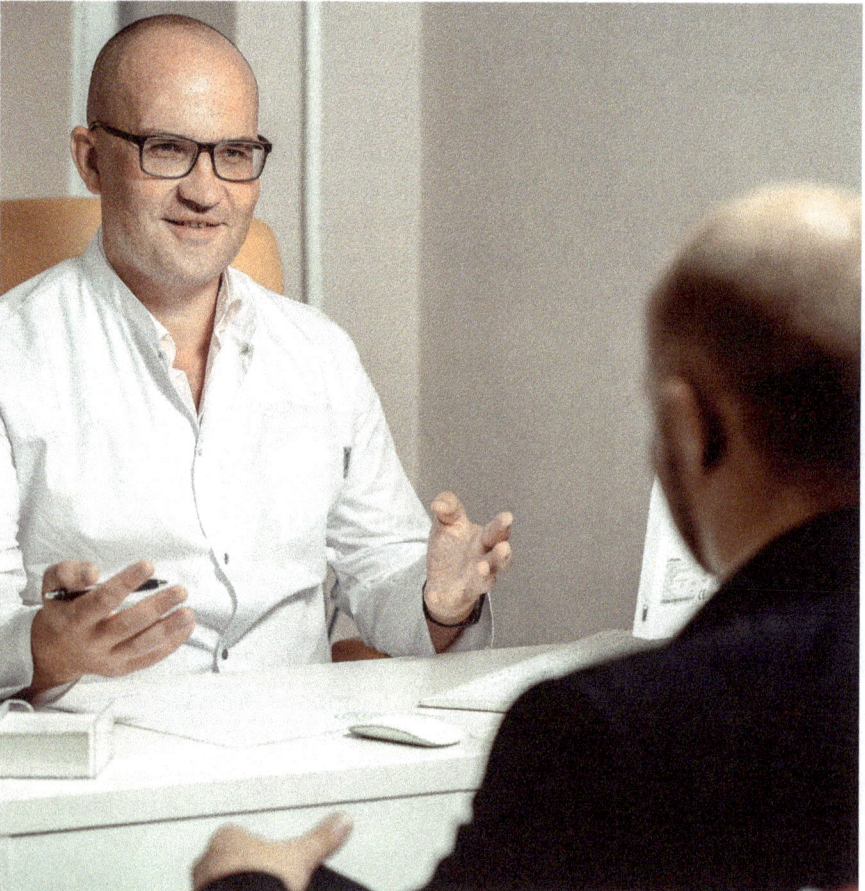

SCREENING FOR OTHER PSYCHIATRIC DISORDERS

The health care professional will also conduct a thorough review to know if the person has other psychiatric disorders similar to ADHD, or those that coexist with ADHD. ADHD regularly coexists with other symptoms like depression, anxiety disorders, learning disabilities, and drug use disorders. The symptoms of these conditions are similar to those of ADHD and may be mistaken for it.

Therefore, a comprehensive evaluation has to thoroughly check for coexisting conditions. If other conditions are detected alongside ADHD, they should all be diagnosed and treated. Treatment for ADHD often fails when the coexisting conditions remain untreated. It is important to confirm that ADHD is not a secondary consequence of anxiety, depression, or other psychiatric disorders to ensure effective treatment.

The person will need to answer questions focusing on their health history going as far back as early childhood, including drug and alcohol abuse, academic and work experience, family life, marital life, and social history. The health professional will also try to identify patterns specific to people with ADHD and figure out if they are caused by other disorders.

Family Participation

Before a complete diagnosis of ADHD, a close relation needs to be interviewed. This could be a spouse, parent, sibling, partner, or any other close-knit person. This procedure is done to collate more information. It is common for most adults with ADHD to have troubles recollecting their past, especially from childhood, and so may not remember past diagnoses or details. This prompts the health professional to request that their parents/guardians fill out a retrospective ADHD profile describing childhood behavior.

Some adults with ADHD are unaware of the extent of the problems their ADHD behaviors cause for them, as well as the impact on others. For married or cohabiting couples, a joint interview to review the ADHD symptoms is beneficial. Doing this will help the non-ADHD spouse or partner have a deeper understanding of how their ADHD partner's symptoms have affected the relationship. This helps them develop empathy for their partner and creates a pathway for the improvement of the relationship. The health care professional can get those loved ones to fill checklists of symptoms if they cannot be part of the interviews.

The entire process of evaluation for an adult with ADHD can be frustrating and embarrassing. However, this should not prevent the person with ADHD from opening up about their symptoms or feeling ashamed. The diagnosis and treatment of the individual with ADHD heavily depends on how accurate the information they provide is.

Standardized Behavior Rating Scales

There should be one or more standardized behavior rating scales in a comprehensive evaluation. Questionnaires are created based on research to compare the behavior of people with ADHD to those of people without ADHD. Whatever scores gotten on the rating scales do not serve as a diagnosis, but they are necessary to provide objective information for the evaluation process. The rating scales are often completed by the person with ADHD and their loved one.

Extra Tests

The health professional may recommend extra psychological, neuropsychological, or learning disabilities tests based on the nature of the disorder being treated. The tests may not indicate ADHD directly, but will provide more information on the effects of ADHD on the individual. These tests will help the professional determine if there are coexisting conditions. For instance, a test of intellectual ability may be required to detect any learning disabilities.

Medical Examination

The health professional may advise a physical exam to ensure the symptoms are not a result of medical issues, especially if the person has not done one in the last six months. The medical examination is necessary for ruling out the presence of other problems or conditions, but is not exactly a confirmation for ADHD.

CONCLUSION OF THE EVALUATION

To end the evaluation, the clinician will compile all of the information obtained from many sources, write a report, and give diagnostic opinions regarding the ADHD condition and other possible disorders that may have been discovered during the evaluation. The health professional will then suggest treatment options and help the person in creating a course of the right medical treatment plans. The health care professional will then forward their findings and proposed treatment plans to the person's primary care providers.

CHAPTER 2

TREATMENT OF ADHD

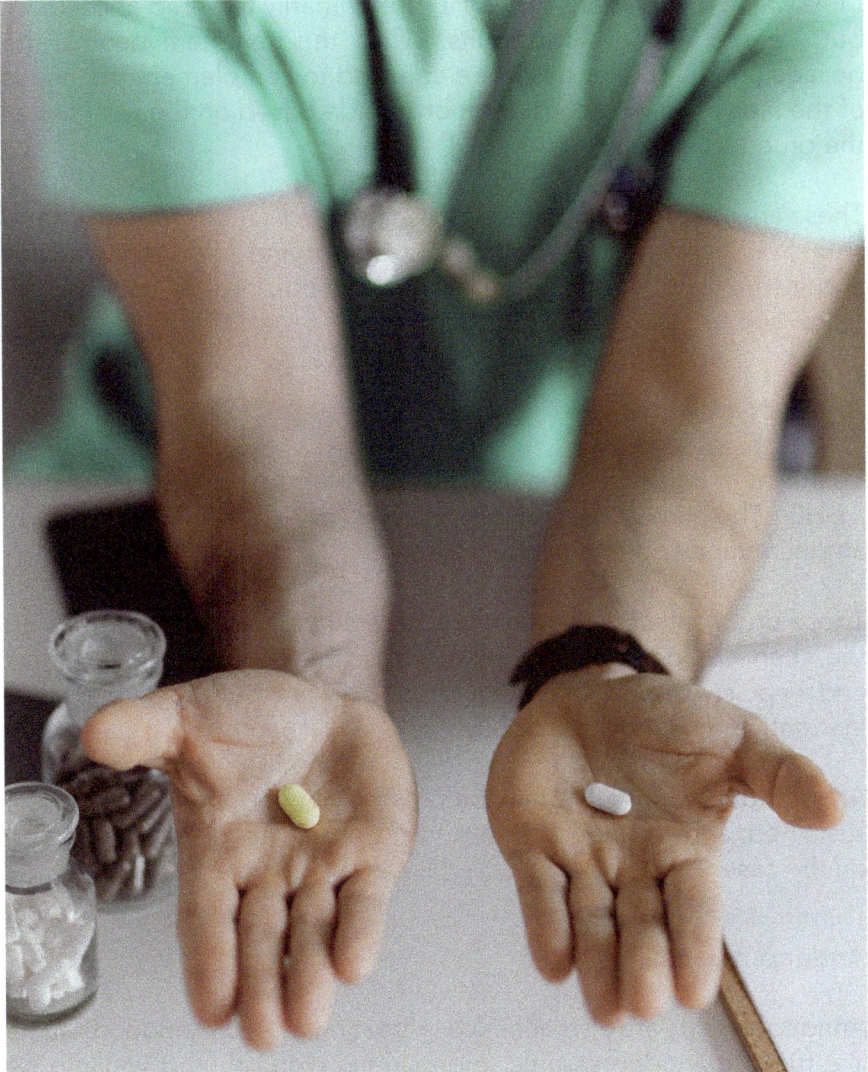

ADHD treatment is quite complicated and has to be created to suit each person. There are different treatment methods that can be considered. Although medication works faster, it is not effective when used alone. Additional treatment includes educational programs, behavioral management, psychological counseling, and family support.

MEDICATIONS FOR ADHD

Most of the medications for ADHD are primarily targeted at children, but are also effective for adults. When the treatment begins, the dosage and frequency has to be adjusted to complement the needs of the individual with considerations made based on the qualities of the drug.

These are the group of drugs classified as medications for ADHD and you should always consult with your doctor and follow their advice and instructions. You should never take medicines on your own or follow someone else's prescription.

Psychostimulants

Stimulant medications are the most preferred option for treating ADHD. The stimulants commonly used for treating ADHD include amphetamine and methylphenidate.

These drugs affect the neurotransmitters responsible for producing the chemical 'dopamine.' These drugs usually reduce Hyperactive and Impulsive behaviors in children, but can be effective against Inattentive type ADHD in adults.

An individual with ADHD may be prescribed with immediate release, sustained, and extended-release forms of the stimulants depending on the case.

Antidepressants

Antidepressants are also effective in treating ADHD. Antidepressants like tricyclic antidepressants, monoamine oxidase, and venlafaxine are usually prescribed. Although the FDA has not approved antidepressants for ADHD use, some doctors still prescribe them, especially in cases where ADHD coexists with depression.

Non-Stimulants

Non-stimulants are medications used for individuals with ADHD who have no response to stimulants or react negatively to them. The drugs are also prescribed for those who have coexisting conditions. Non-stimulants for ADHD include atomoxetine and guanfacine.

SIDE EFFECTS OF ADHD DRUGS

Using ADHD drugs may trigger side effects like
- poor appetite
- headaches
- abdominal pain
- anxiety
- sleep disturbances

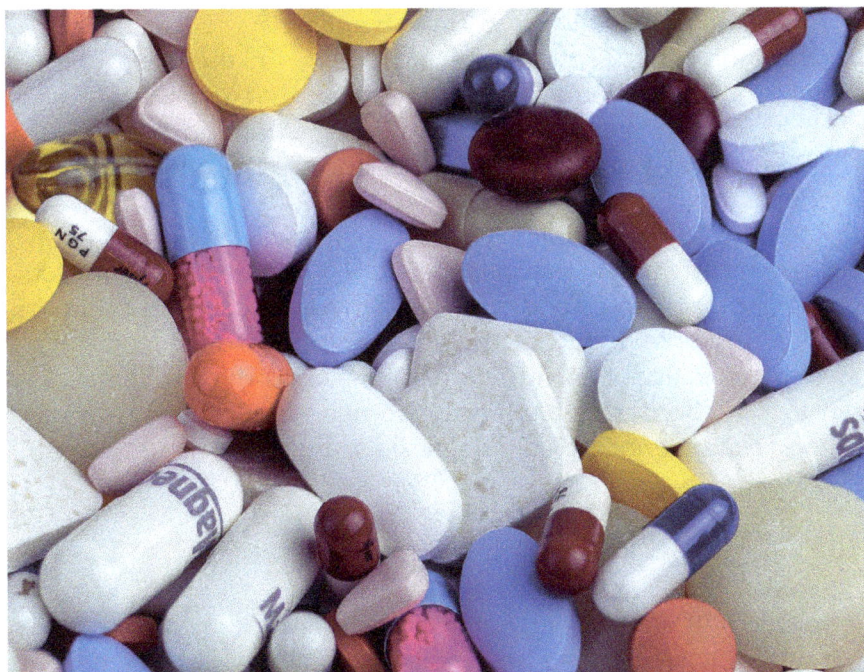

THERAPY AND OTHER BEHAVIORAL TREATMENTS

Adults with ADHD will need therapy and other behavioral treatments in addition to their medications. This is necessary to deal with daily stressors. Medication affects the body's neurological system and the brain, while behavior therapy deals with particular problem behaviors the individual has. The person learns how to structure their time, build routines, and boost positive outcomes.

These other treatment methods are focused on reconditioning the behavior of adults with ADHD, and are listed below.

Cognitive Behavioral Therapy (CBT)

CBT is usually combined with medication. The person with ADHD works together with a therapist to identify problem behaviors and create working methods to make them better. CBT is a temporary, goal-focused type of psychotherapy that works by transforming the individual's negative thoughts and feelings.

This is the process:
1. One problem behavior is corrected at a time.
2. The individual discovers the motivation for the behavior and transforms the thoughts and perceptions that fuel it.
3. They work on practical ways to reform the behavior.
4. They try out the strategies and switch to new ones if they are ineffective.

CBT is great for many individuals with ADHD. People who do not cope with CBT are exempted and often need more structured approaches, especially people with the oppositional defiant disorder who are uncooperative about changing their behaviors. The CBT process of transforming distorted thoughts to reform behavior patterns can also be used to treat mood disorders, anxiety, and other similar issues.

Relaxation Techniques

People with ADHD can find relief from their symptoms by practicing relaxation techniques like yoga and meditation. These techniques relax the mind and body while also focusing on the individual's thoughts.

Practicing meditation for a long time helps people manage their emotions better. People with ADHD can improve their attention span, which allows them to work through situations.

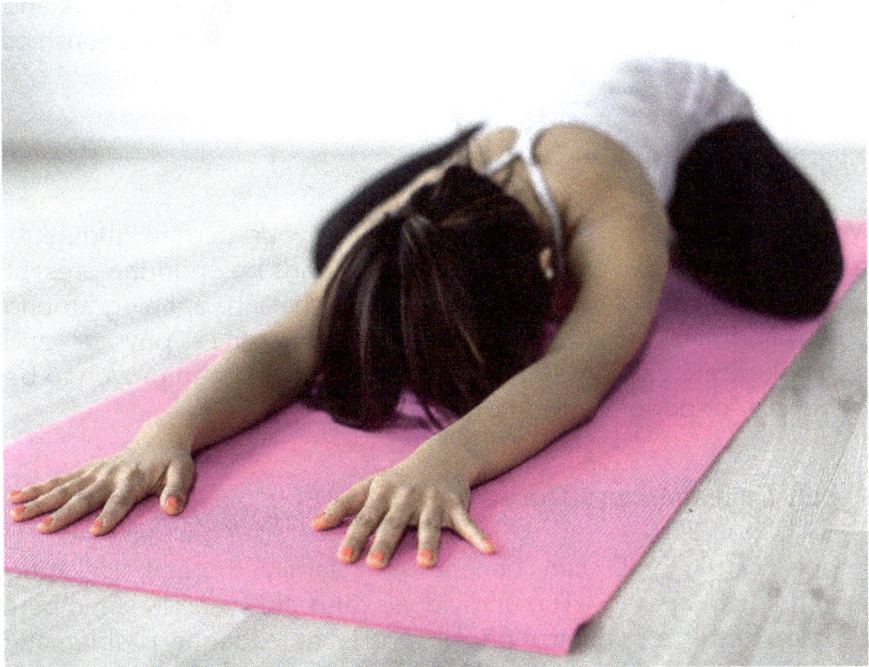

Coaching

People with ADHD can benefit from life or job coaching. Coaching is a new treatment approach where people with ADHD work closely with coaches who help them:

- Create structures for planning their lives and dealing with daily challenges through feedback, recommendations, and encouragement.
- Set and achieve goals.
- Improve time and money management skills.
- Stay motivated.

Coaches help individuals to generally improve their lives by taking on the responsibilities of a teacher, cheerleader, taskmaster, and personal assistant.

People using coaches can schedule weekly meetings. This may mean frequent phone meetings. In some cases, the coaches visit their clients' homes to assist with their social or organizational skills. Using coaches helps people with ADHD improve organization at work and progress at their jobs. It also helps them improve their relationships at home.

Mindful Meditation

Mindful awareness means centering on your current thoughts, feelings, and body sensations. It simply means being in the present and being incredibly aware of everything that's happening around you. Mindfulness can be used to improve one's physical and psychological health. Mindfulness exercises have been proven to be beneficial for people with ADHD.

Family Education and Therapy

People with ADHD can benefit from family therapy, including marriage counseling. The individuals and their family members develop better communication skills and learn to identify problematic patterns. Counseling helps the family understand that the person with ADHD is not deliberately messy or forgetful, and their problem goes beyond that.

E-Therapy

People who find conventional therapists expensive, cannot access qualified professionals in their area, or feel uncomfortable having a personal visit with a doctor can opt for e-therapy. E-therapy is conducted in several ways.

Phone Calls

Phone counseling has been around for a while. Therapists who have used this method have positive reviews about it. The therapists and the individuals with ADHD discuss over the phone. This option is great because it is

- affordable
- very convenient
- anonymous
- provides a higher sense of control for the individual with ADHD

Video Conferencing

Video conferencing is great for individuals living in rural areas who might be unable to travel or access qualified professionals. This session is more frequent than one-on-one counseling.

Text-Based Communication

People can also access therapists easily via email, chat rooms, or direct messages. This form of therapy is new but has some evidence backing its effectiveness.

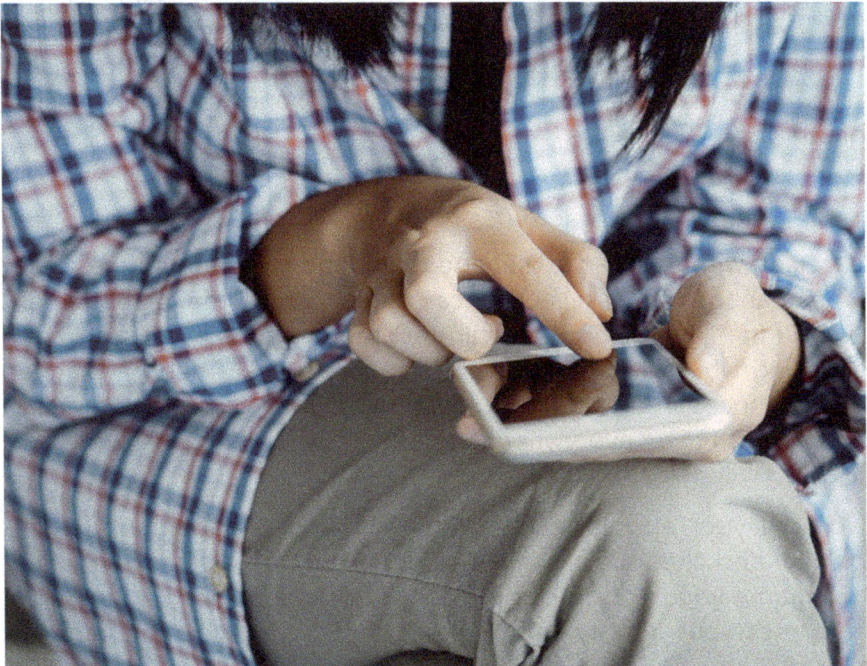

MANAGING ADHD SYMPTOMS: BEHAVIORAL STRATEGIES

People with ADHD have trouble dealing with work, relationships, organization, and other tasks. Besides medications and other treatment plans, there are different lifestyle changes that people with ADHD can embrace to improve their symptoms and regain control of their life. Many of the changes might seem tedious initially, but consistently making them a habit will improve your life. Here are some behavioral strategies.

Getting Organized

People with ADHD have difficulties organizing things either at work or at home. To help manage ADHD, it is necessary to create a realistic organization strategy that works long-term. A well-organized space allows for ease in carrying out several activities, lowers anxiety, boosts efficiency, and lowers pressure on relationships. Practice organization using these strategies.

Learn to Declutter

Things will be better organized if there's little clutter, as it helps you know what point to start organizing from. Start from the easiest part of the junk because it helps to break down the large task into smaller sizes. Also, try to get everything needed handy before you start organizing.

Time Management

A person with ADHD can manage their condition better if they learn time management skills. You can boost your time management skills in many ways, and you can test the methods available before choosing what will work for you. For starters, you need a planner. Your planner can be a notebook or an app. Make sure it's something that you can carry everywhere.

Note all your appointments, meetings, and engagements in the planner and check it daily. When you have a task, overestimate how much time you need to complete it. You can add ten minutes extra and track your activity with a watch rather than your phone. This

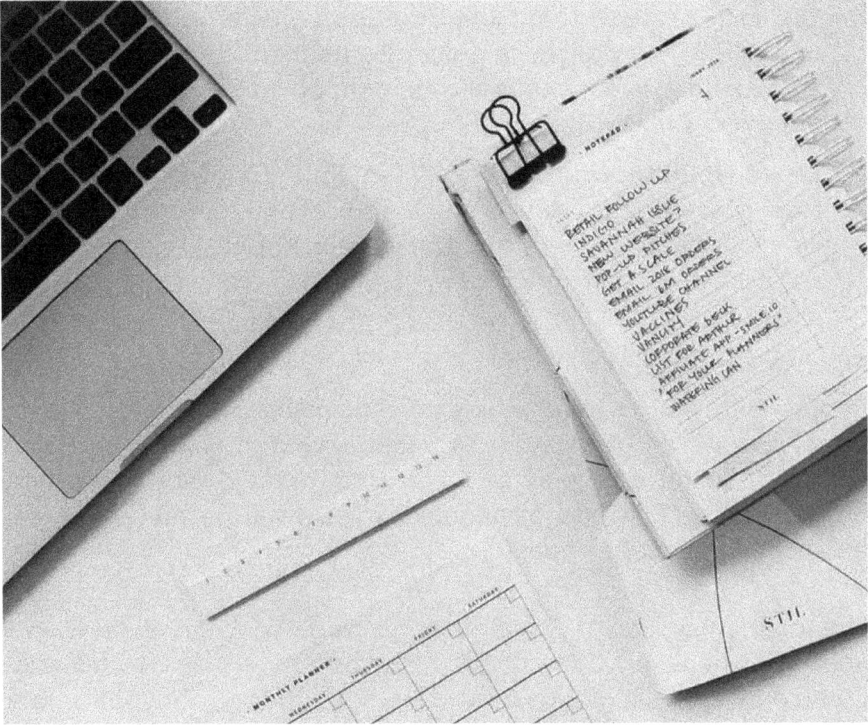

helps you track the time without distractions. Start a routine; you'll be more organized if you create a routine. This helps you keep to your tasks at the scheduled time.

Task Management

Besides your space, other areas of your life need organization, too. Individuals with ADHD also have trouble organizing work or school tasks. Do these to help you organize your tasks and stay updated:

- **Have a list:** When you check your planner daily, note down the tasks for the day. Arrange these tasks in order of priority, especially based on time sensitivity. Work through the tasks according to your arrangement.

- **Divide big projects:** When you divide your big projects into smaller tasks, it helps you manage them easily. Increase the amount of projects you're handling as you progress. The problem is usually about starting and keeping your focus on the project.

You can create a 15-minute time loop where you concentrate entirely on your project for a start. If after then, you think you need a break, take five minutes and go right on into work immediately after your break.

- **Leave multitasking aside:** When you concentrate on one task at a time, you will improve your overall productivity. With concentration, you're sure to achieve 100 percent on one task rather than 50 percent on 5.

Finance Management

People with ADHD have problems with managing money due to behaviors like impulsivity, procrastination, or disorganization. Being proactive is the best way to keep your money habits in check. Set reminders. Bills and payment deadlines will be met if you set reminders on your calendar.

Use online banking. With online banking, you can access your accounts whenever you want, allowing you to make payments easily. Some online banking apps provide budgeting tools for you to track your expenses.

Driving

Most people have trouble concentrating while driving, but this is a very serious problem for adults with ADHD. While you drive, it is best to learn how distractions can affect you. Remove things that can cause distractions, like phones.

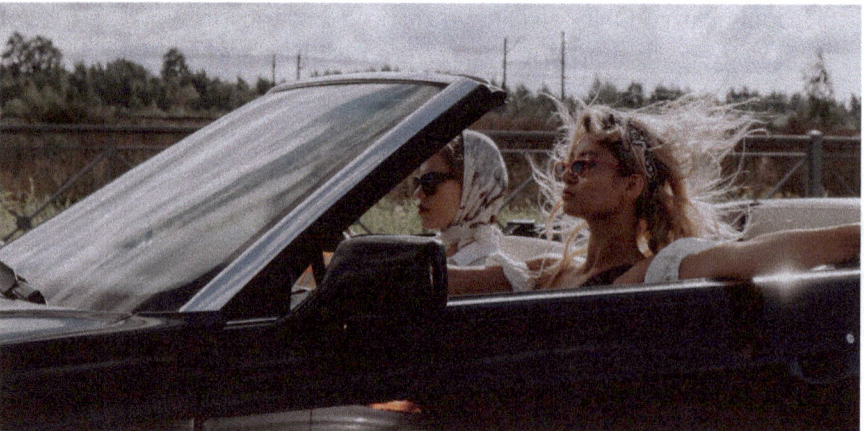

NATURAL WAYS TO MANAGE ADHD

In the search for treatment for ADHD, you can choose to use natural strategies. The following natural ways of relieving ADHD can be used with or without medication.

- **Consume nutrient-rich and whole foods:** Foods rich in protein, omega-3, and other nutrients, including low-processed grains, are a source of energy for adults and children. They improve the brain and support neurotransmitter function.

  → Neurotransmitters transport neural signals across the brain and body and hugely regulate attention, concentration, as well as processing of information.

  → Consuming nutrient-rich meals and balanced diets will provide the energy needed for adequate functioning of the body's neurotransmitters. This helps in reducing ADHD symptoms.

- **Stay away from sensitive food:** Having a food sensitivity or intolerance can increase your chances of having a leaky gut and intestinal inflammation. The effect of this on your gut bacteria and production of neurotransmitters is unpleasant, thereby aggravating the symptoms of aggression and impulsivity.

  → You can use tests to find out your sensitivities, but people are usually triggered by gluten or dairy. When wheat or dairy are improperly digested, particles are found in the urine. These particles in the urine have been linked to ADHD. If you have been diagnosed with ADHD, you might want to get gluten and/or dairy out of your meals for a minimum of six weeks, even if you are not sensitive.

- **Clear nutrient deficiencies:** ADHD has a connection to several nutrient deficiencies, like vitamins B-complex, magnesium, omega-3 fatty acids, and zinc. These nutrients are often complementary to each other and having a deficiency in any of them can cause malfunctioning of the others.

  → A combination of magnesium supplements and vitamin B6 has been shown to boost magnesium absorption, which can lower ADHD symptoms.

- **Treat your leaky gut:** Your gut is important for the proper functioning of your body. In the gut, good bacteria reside and produce important neurotransmitters, such as dopamine and serotonin, while absorbing nutrients like vitamin B-complex and magnesium. If you fix your gut, you will have fewer gastrointestinal symptoms and notice an improvement in your attention span, mood, and general health.

  → If you constantly deal with constipation, food sensitivity, bloating, sugar cravings, or problems with your bowel movements, then you probably need to get your gut checked.

- **Boost antioxidant levels:** Constant exposure to free radicals can affect DNA structure, brain, and important body cells. Free radicals are unstable and harmful. Antioxidants stabilize free radicals and prevent oxidative damage. Consume antioxidants like vitamin C and glutathione to increase the amount of antioxidants in your body.

- **Detoxify your body:** Exposure to heavy metals is harmful to the body's neurodevelopmental functions, and produces toxins that are problematic to cognitive function. As a result, heavy metals are linked to the onset of ADHD. Children who are genetically prone to ADHD can develop the condition if overexposed to heavy metals. People with ADHD usually do not have great detoxification systems. Detoxifying the body will help reduce symptoms of ADHD.

- **Reduce excitotoxins:** Excitotoxins are materials that excessively trigger neuron receptors. Neuron receptors assist brain cell communication and work faster than usual when they are exposed to excitotoxins. When this happens, the individual can experience impulsivity, hyperactivity, and problems with concentration.

  → Artificial food additives like FD&C yellow, aspartame, MSG, or glutamates are regarded as excitotoxins and should be avoided.

- **Have a steady sleep routine:** People with ADHD experience an improvement in concentration, attention, and energy when they have regular, satisfying sleep.

→ As a result of their symptoms, they often have sleep problems and wake up tired or grumpy. This further aggravates the ADHD symptoms and exacerbates the sleep problems in a vicious cycle. However, people with ADHD can find relief if they create a healthy night time routine. A sleep routine makes sleep easier and contributes to reducing the ADHD symptoms.

• **Reduce screen time:** Individuals with ADHD have higher chances of being addicted to the internet. From research, around 25 percent of people with the disorder also deal with internet addiction (Love, 2020). When people are exposed to more screen time, their ADHD symptoms worsen. Although the connection between the two is vague, it is still not advised. Increasing screen time — especially before bed — puts everyone at risk of having sleep problems.

→ Therefore, a person with ADHD may see a reduction in symptoms if they minimize screen time and sleep more.

• **Exercise:** People with ADHD will experience a marked difference in their symptoms if they exercise. Exercise causes some improvement in certain areas of cognitive performance (Stieg, 2019). Both individuals with and those without benefit from exercise, as the research reports faster speed in processing and inhibitory control in the two groups.

• **Increase caffeine consumption:** Stimulants are among the important ADHD medications. This means a person with ADHD can get relief from tea or coffee. Consuming caffeine can reduce inattention and relieve the Hyperactivity-Impulsivity symptoms. People with ADHD who drink regular coffee may notice that their symptoms increase when they stop.

→ Caffeine consumption boosts concentration, brain function, and responsiveness in individuals. It is a very efficient tool for building working memory. However, regular consumption of caffeine may cause some level of nervousness for people without ADHD, while reducing the symptoms in people with ADHD. However, before you go right into coffee as a stimulant, ensure your doctor confirms it's safe for you.

OVERCOMING ADHD PROBLEMS IN REAL LIFE

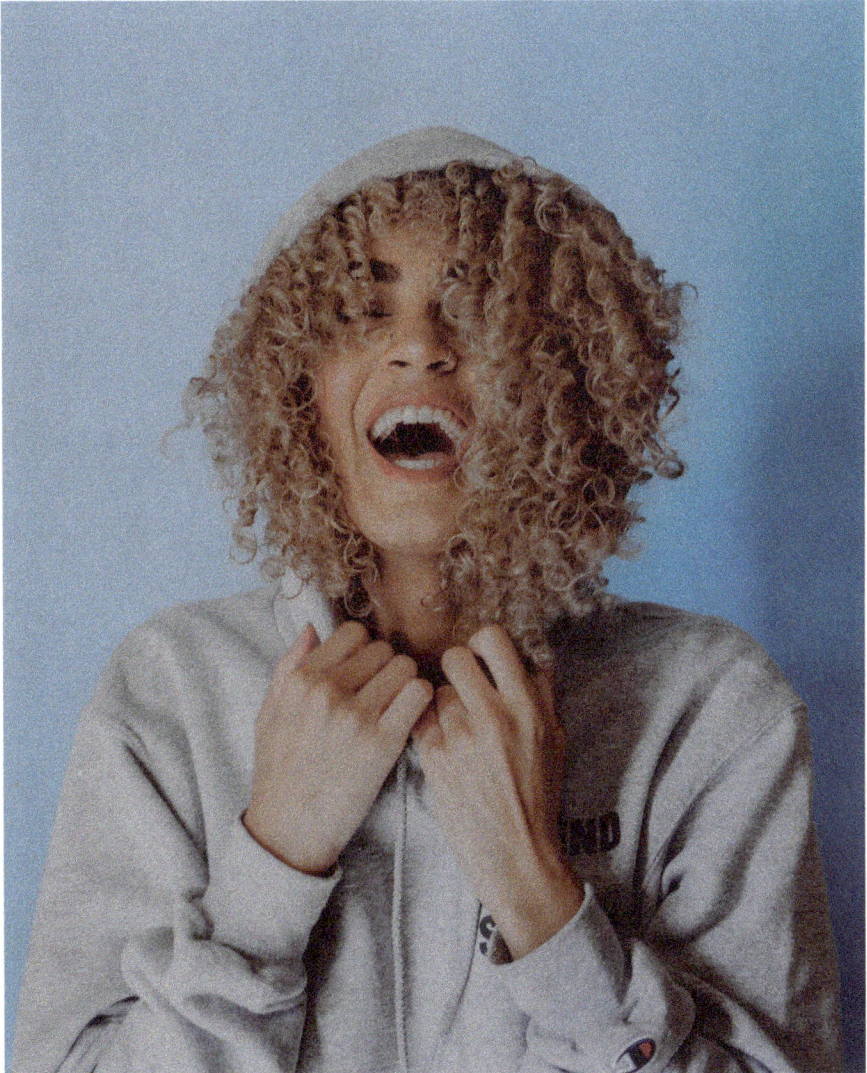

SUCCEEDING AT WORK

Living with Attention Deficit Hyperactive Disorder can be complicated for most adults. While some individuals with the disorder are able to navigate their way around it and develop high ranking careers, others struggle with many challenges. Many people with this disorder suffer from communication problems, are easily distracted, become procrastinators, and struggle with sophisticated projects.

But all hope isn't lost for those with ADHD. These are some ways to manage these struggles and build a better work life.

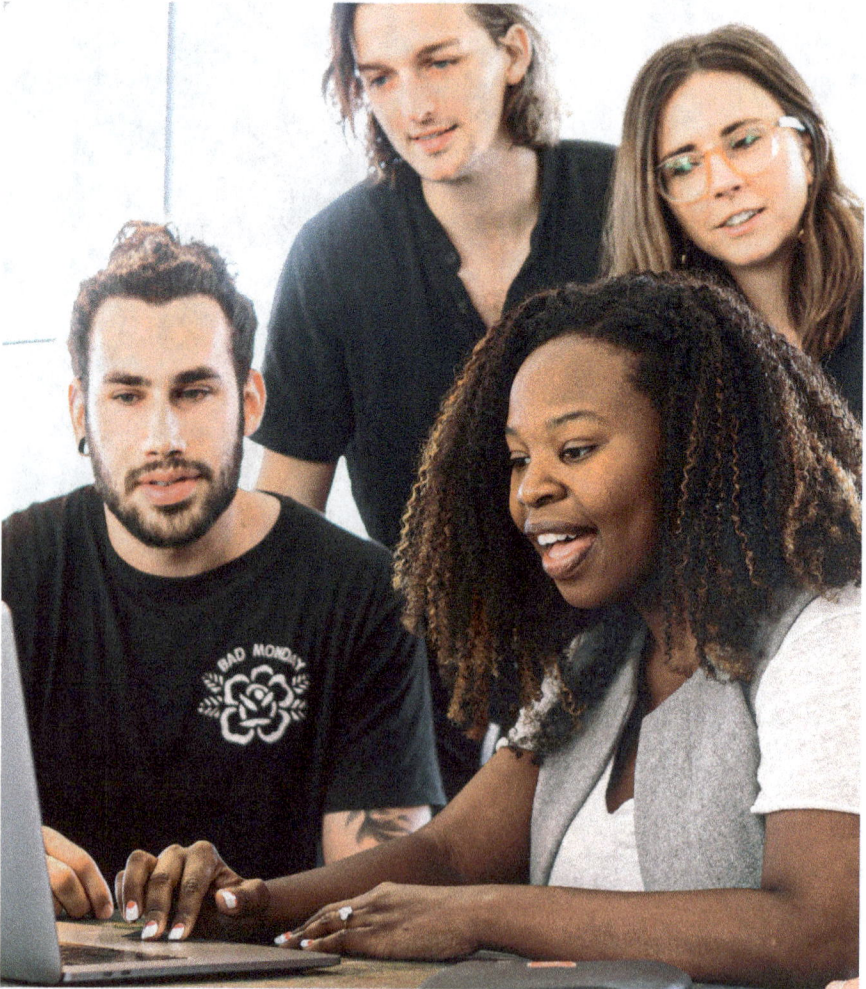

Getting Easily Distracted

People with ADHD struggle with internal and external distractions. The external distractions arise from noises or disturbances in the working environment, while internal distractions occur within the psyche of the individual, like daydreams.

→ **How to manage:** Using noise cancelling headphones during work can reduce external sounds. You can close your office door if possible to prevent distraction from colleagues. Stay off social media if there is an urgent task to accomplish. Having a to-do list can improve focus on current tasks and reduce the urge to daydream.

Impulsivity

During moments of frustration, people with ADHD may become bad tempered and impulsive.

→ **How to manage:** Find out your triggers and learn different, more appropriate ways to channel your frustration. You can work with a coach, practice mindfulness and self-talk, or get constructive feedback from people around to discover those triggers.

Hyperactivity

Fidgeting and trouble sitting still are one of the many symptoms of ADHD.

→ **How to manage:** Choose jobs that allow frequent movement and activity. People with ADHD do well as teachers, salespeople, and exercise trainers. If you are already in a more static job, take regular breaks, jot vital facts during meetings, and move easily. You might want to come to work with your lunch rather than buying, so the free time can be channeled towards exercising.

Poor Memory

People with ADHD perform poorly at their jobs when they cannot meet deadlines or follow project instructions.

→ **How to manage:** Bring recording devices to work to record instructions, place complicated tasks into checklists, and use sticky notes to help with memory.

Boredom Blockouts

People with ADHD fall into boredom easily, especially when handling routine tasks or tedious paperwork.

→ **How to manage:** Fight boredom by using a timer to keep you on your tasks, categorizing bulky tasks into smaller ones, taking frequent breaks, or getting a more stimulating job.

Time Management

People with ADHD have problems keeping to time. In many cases, they perform tasks without noting the amount of time spent on it. How to manage: Split up your tasks into smaller parts with different deadlines. When you meet a deadline, reward yourself. Have reminders for meetings and important tasks.

Procrastination

Adults procrastinate sometimes, but it is almost an identity for people with ADHD.

→ **How to manage:** Divide big projects into smaller tasks, get the supervisor to monitor task deadlines, and partner with a time efficient colleague if possible.

Paperwork/Details

Job performance will drop drastically if a person cannot locate important documents, submit reports and time sheets, and manage a filing system.

→ **How to manage:** Set up a filing system or delegate paperwork tasks to an administrative assistant, and discard unwanted papers regularly.

Interpersonal/Social Skills

People with ADHD may get on their colleagues' nerves unintentionally due to frequent interruption, being talkative, not listening properly, or being too blunt.

→ **How to manage:** Study social cues, request for feedback from people around, practice with a coach, or find a job position where you have less interaction with others.

Difficulty Managing Long-Term Projects

One of the hardest work functions that people with ADHD struggle with is managing long-term projects due to struggles with time management, arranging materials, monitoring progress, and sharing successes.

→ **How to manage:** Divide long term projects into smaller parts so they can be easy to handle, reduce the time duration for the projects to take advantage of 'sprinting' abilities, pair up with a colleague, and/or find jobs that need short term tasks only if it is impossible to manage long term projects.

SUCCEEDING IN LIFE

Success is relative, but there are things and achievements generally applauded, like meeting all our life goals, sustaining healthy relationships, and excelling in our chosen career. People with ADHD often struggle to meet these standards, especially when their symptoms are in conflict with their efforts.

A person can only fix a problem when they know where the challenge is. After getting a diagnosis, it is necessary to work with a specialist and identify ways in which the symptoms affect one's life. The specialist can formulate treatment plans to change the problematic sectors of their life.

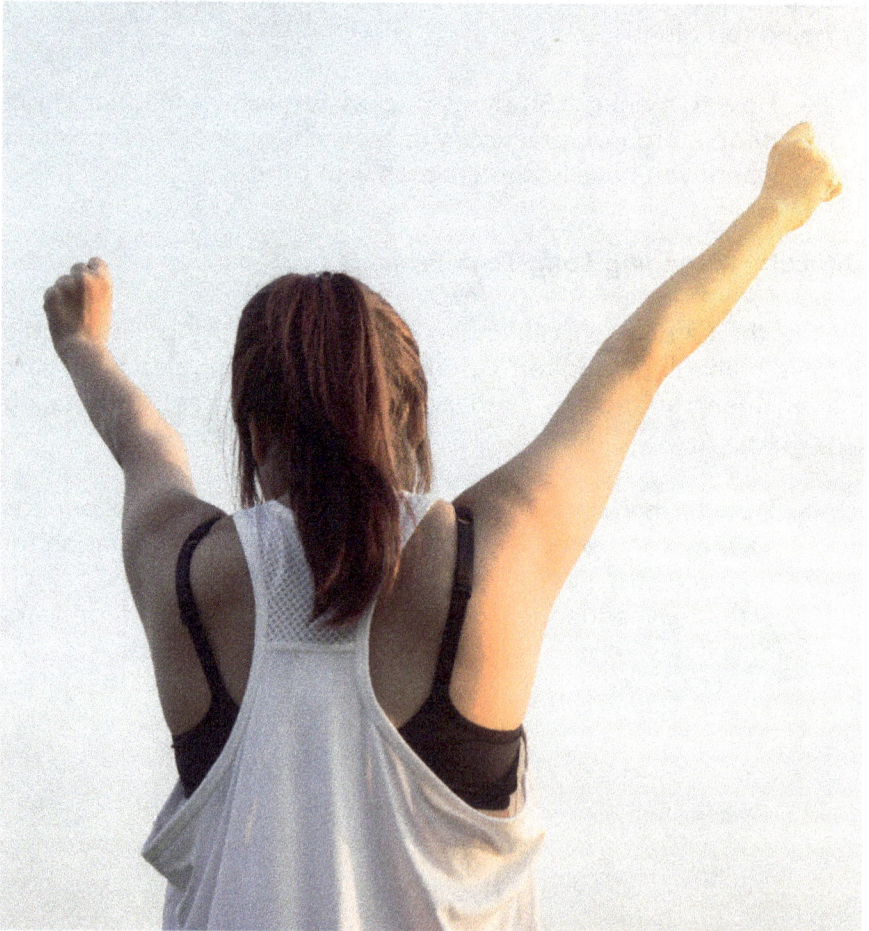

Here are some ways to achieve success in the areas of life that matter to you.

Personal Life

- **Be orderly:** You can maintain orderliness in your home or office if you work with a friend, or use a self-help book or website. ADHD affects brain functions and people with the disorder cannot organize information. As a result, they struggle with keeping up with basic information, like mail and other home tasks.

- **Delegate tasks:** Don't feel shy to get a virtual assistant or employ a home cleaning service. Link your bank accounts to an automated bill pay system. Join friends or family members to make holiday dinners. Get someone to help you out with your tasks if your symptoms prevent you from completing them.

- **Reduce your commitments:** People with ADHD often take up commitments due to impulsivity. Check your calendar, analyze your lifestyle, and notice where you are spending your energy. Reduce the tasks to those that are most rewarding.

Social Life

- **Set up a working calendar and email system:** Put reminders for important events, like anniversaries, birthdays, family outings. Find one day to send out greeting cards instead of doing them at different times.

- **Have a pocket notebook or use a notebook app:** Write down the ideas you have or things you need to say in conversations. This prevents you from interrupting or branching out conversations into unwanted directions. It also helps you take note of cool ideas before you forget them.

- **Inform a friend or family member:** If those around you know what you struggle with, they can cue you privately in social events if you're neglecting social cues or dominating a conversation.

SUCCEEDING IN RELATIONSHIPS

People with ADHD struggle with maintaining relationships. However, you can build a successful relationship with the right practices. These are some things to do to prevent your symptoms from influencing your relationship.

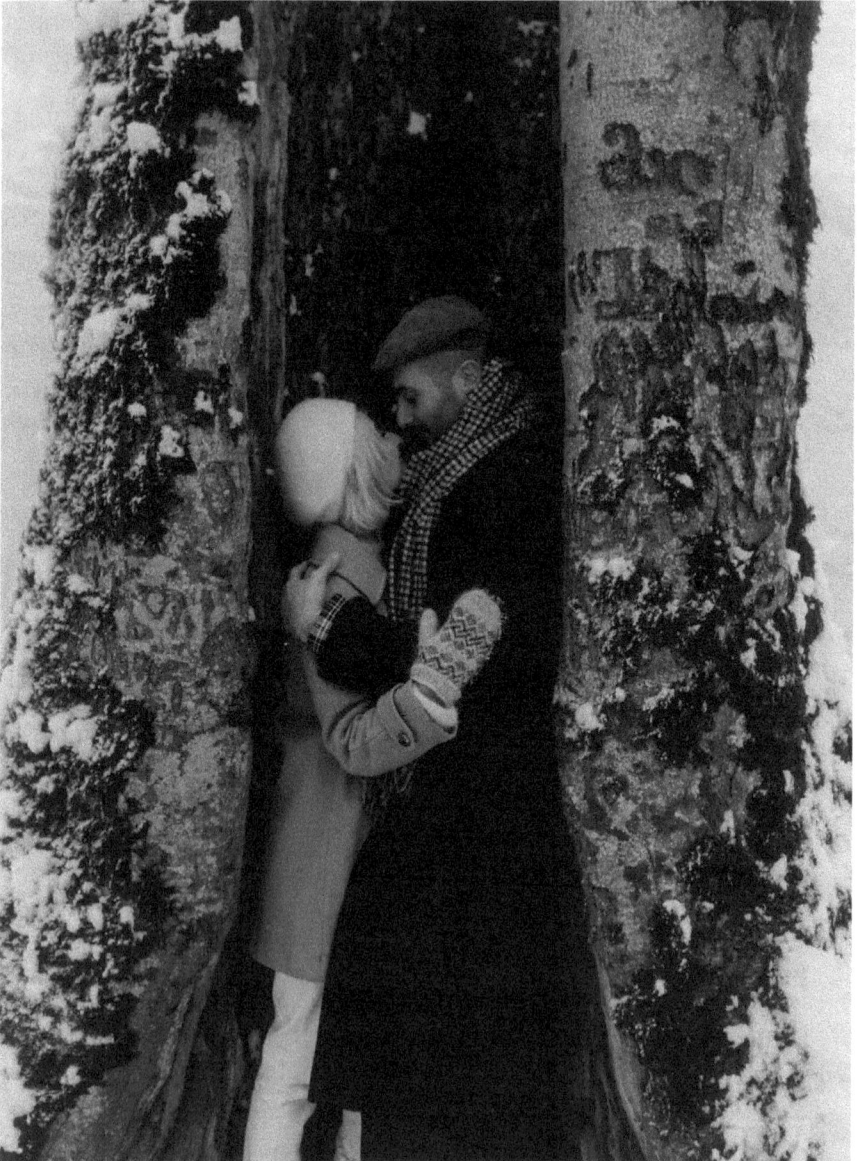

- **Cooperate with your physician for an efficient treatment plan:** This strategy involves getting a correct diagnosis. People with ADHD often have coexisting conditions that can impact their life and relationship. Ensure that you are using a treatment plan that works with an accurate diagnosis.

- **Utilize the positive ADHD characteristics:** Rather than focusing on the negative, boost your relationship with your positive characteristics like creativity, spontaneity, energy bursts, and problem solving skills. Your partner probably fell in love with these characteristics. Remember why your partner is attracted to you and let this guide you. If you think about the positive characteristics that you both contribute to the relationship, it becomes easy to deal with other struggles.

- **Discuss ADHD with your partner:** Tell your partner what aspect of ADHD you struggle with, as well as ways in which they can help. If your partner has ADHD, tell them which parts of their symptoms affect you the most. Discuss ADHD with your partner and find coping strategies for problematic symptoms.

- **Identify behaviors that need changing:** If you have ADHD, tell your partner to help you work on a behavior that may be troubling the relationship. Open up about the behavior causing the most difficulty and you and your partner can find solutions to it.

- **Maintain an open communication line:** Be honest and open during communication with your partner regardless of the communication method. Some couples communicate better on the phone. For others, the best time is at night when there are no distractions from any source, including children. And some others are better off dropping notes or going out somewhere together. Find what works for you and your partner and connect as often as you can.

- **Utilize the kitchen calendar:** Put your kitchen calendar to good use. Check it every day to ensure that you are not missing out on details that are important to your partner.

- **Get a chalkboard or whiteboard for seamless communication:** If you feel like you and your partner are just crossing paths around the house, write your thoughts on a board. On days when you might be too busy to connect, put down notes to remind them or yourself of tasks that need completion.

- **Share household chores based on individual strengths:** You don't have to stick to traditional roles. Share chores based on your capabilities. Let chores that need excessive movement be assigned to the partner who has a problem sitting still. Sharing chores based on strengths will increase the chances of completion.

- **Notice the positives:** Shower sincere compliments on your spouse regularly. Applaud them for the things they are doing well. This way they understand that you see and appreciate their effort. It might be awkward to offer compliments initially, but as you get used to it, it feels more natural and your partner can also respond positively.

- **Create time to spend together:** Go on evening dates. If you have kids, get someone to watch them and go do fun things with your partner. List out several activities that you both enjoy and find time to do them. Let your partner know that you want to partake in the activities that they like because you want to share their company. Enjoy the time you spend with each other.

DEVELOPING ORGANIZATIONAL SKILLS

People with ADHD struggle with organizing. At first, it is hard to start, but you can reward yourself to boost motivation to be more organized. If you want to get better at organizing, start by putting your house in order. Provide rewards for yourself for when you finish the tasks.

You can ease the task by asking for help from a friend. This comes in handy if you need to declutter. Your friend helps you discard unwanted items because they do not have sentimental connections to them. Find support in online chat groups. You can join those that have features which allow you to set commitments to organize a space, then you step away from your computer to organize, and eventually come back to motivate others.

Organizing with a timer and music helps you work. You can set your timer at 15-minute intervals and have breaks in between. Creating a music playlist to keep you company while you work is also a good idea.

A Working Strategy to Build Organizational Skills

As earlier mentioned, the best method to perform a complex task is to divide it into much smaller tasks and attend to those tasks one at a time. If you have to organize a living space like your house, you can divide the process into these steps:

- Choose the spaces you want to organize.
- Arrange them from the easiest to the hardest.
- Begin with the easiest space.
- Create a time schedule to start organizing.
- Choose a reward or motivation for completing the steps.
- Share the space into sections.
- Organize one section at a time and focus on completing it before moving to another.
- After completing the easiest space, proceed to a harder one and continue.

Choose a Space and Create a Time Schedule

First, you must list out all the physical spaces you want to organize from easiest to hardest. If there are rooms in your house, arrange them in order of cleaning needs. Keep the list somewhere you can have easy access to it. When you choose the easiest space from your list, decide how long it will take to organize it. Set a deadline. Add more time if the estimate is inadequate. Share the estimated time into several short work sessions

.

The time interval should be somewhere between 30–60 minutes. If you easily get bored you can reduce the interval to 10–15 minutes and increase the work sessions. You need to work for short intervals without getting tired or bored. Use a calendar to schedule your activities over a few days and adjust the time estimate if you want.

Split Your Space Into Sections

If you're organizing a house and taking it one room at a time, you might still need to partition the rooms. Split the space (room) into a grid and work on one cell at a time. Here are some ways to partition the space:

- **Quartering:** Divide the space into quarters. If you can't do it visually, use string or masking tape.

- **Clock-based:** Divide the space into different clock-like sections. Stand at one point and mark that spot as 12:00 and start working from there. Move around the room in this manner and map out spots at 1:00, 2:00, 3;00, and so on until you're back at your starting point. If you feel overwhelmed, you can group one or two clock-like sections into a single work session.

- **Zones:** Divide the space sections into zones and seperate the equipment and other items needed in the zone. For instance, if you have to organize your bedroom, your zones can consist of a bed zone, a closet zone, and so on. Ensure everything needed in a zone is placed accordingly.

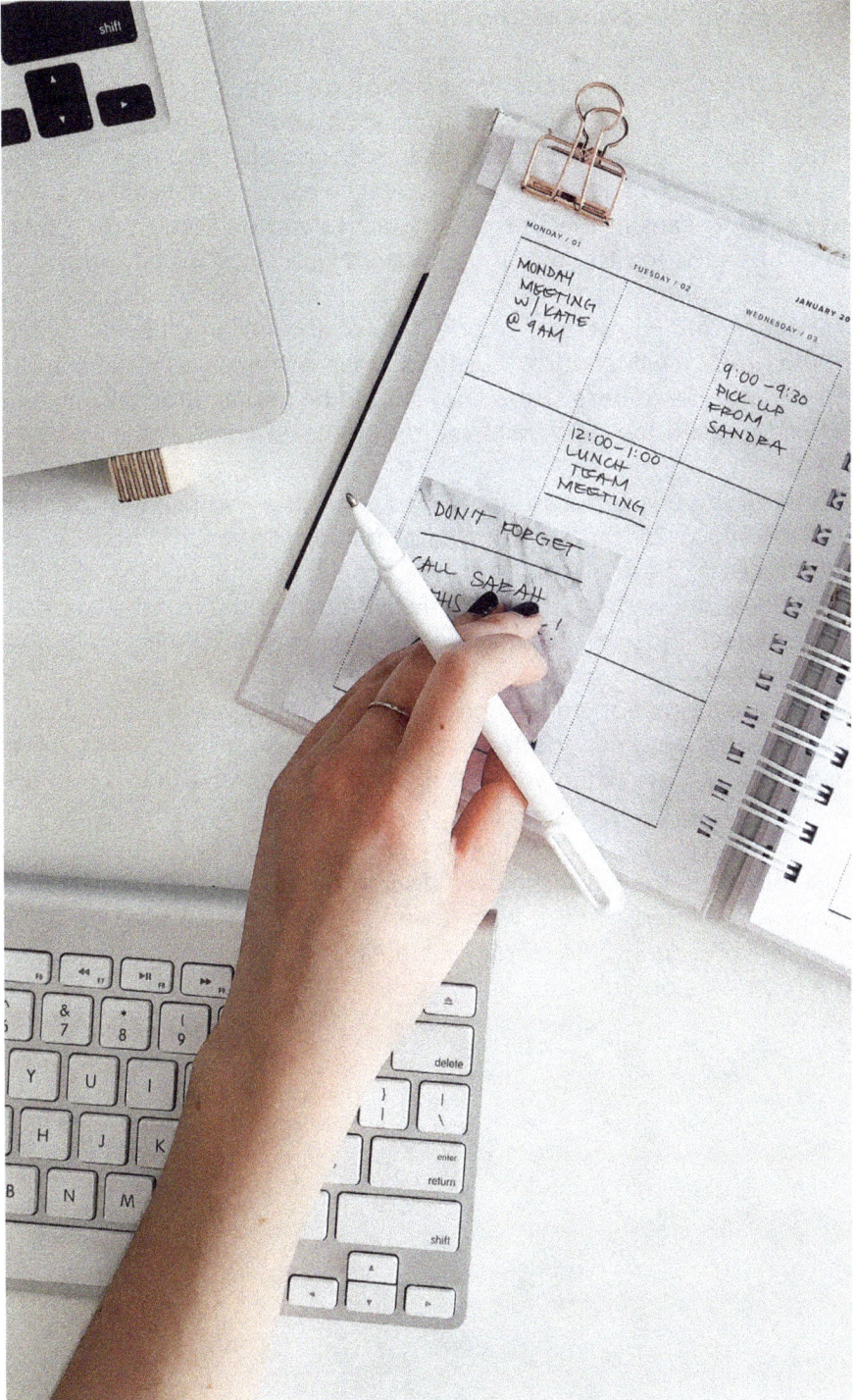

Work on the Sections Methodically

Get all the materials you need, like garbage bags, cleaning supplies, boxes, plastic containers etc., then start your playlist or set your timer. Begin with a trash bag and three boxes labelled, "keep here", "take away," and "not sure" respectively. Throw all leftover food and empty food cans in the trash. Dirty dishes can be kept in the "take away" box for you to drop in the kitchen when you are finished.

For every item you select, decide if it's of any importance and which of the boxes it will go into. If useless, trash it. Items you need should go into the "keep here" box. They should be kept in the "take away" box if they need to be transferred to another section.

Go through your items as fast as you can. When you cannot decide fast to keep or discard an item, store it in the "not sure" box. When your timer or playlist ends, stop the project for the day. Discard the trash. Take the items in the "take away" box to their rightful location even though those places may not yet be organized.

Don't take any action on the "not sure" box until you have completed your sorting. Use masking tape to close the box and indicate on the box a future date when you will open it. This can be in three to six months. Note the opening date on your planner.

When it's time to review the box, discard or give away items that you have not needed since it was sealed. If you have needed an item from the box during the storage time, find the appropriate section of the room to store it.

TIPS TO STAY ORGANIZED

With all the effort you have put into organizing your space, you'll surely want to keep it that way. These are some handy tips to help you prevent clutter.

How to organize paper:
- Recycle or trash it
- Give it away
- Act on it now
- Save or file it

If you have too much paper lying around, consider unsubscribing from mailing lists. You can also take pictures of paper information that you need to save without having the originals; store them on your computer. Arrange the images in computer folders.

Have a Ticker Filing System

If there is regular entry of important papers into your home or office, either through notes, bills, mail, coupons, notes, or phone messages, a ticker filing system becomes necessary. The ticker filing system has dates that help declutter your paperwork. There are 43 folders in the system, one for every month (labeled January–December) and one for every day of the month (labeled 1–31).

Always keep the folder for the current month in front of the 1–31 numbered folders. Ensure the folders are placed in spots you can easily locate. When you get paper, file it in the folder of the date you want to act on it. This system is only effective if you remember to look at the folders every day.

At the beginning of every month, move the folder of the current month to the front and arrange the contents to suit the appropriate dates.

Storage Strategies

Here are some methods to properly store items and keep things organized:

- Store items in clear containers if you're worried you will not find them. Putting them in clear containers helps save time.
- Store certain items in hangers with compartments. These hangers are great for makeup, jewelry, gloves, pantry items, office supplies, tapes or CDs, cleaning supplies, craft supplies, and hats and scarves.
- Keep smaller items in lids and boxes under the bed.
- Get a big trash can to keep spare blankets and sheets and other similar items. Keep the can beside your bed, place a floor length tablecloth over it, and convert it to a night stand.

The launch pad: If you usually spend a lot of time looking for items, create a table or bookshelf by your front door for stuff you need everytime you leave home. Put a small container on the table for you to drop keys, glasses, and wallets. The table can also hold briefcases and backpacks overnight.

Centers: Create centers to store supplies that you need to achieve certain tasks. Keep these items in a mobile container. It helps you save time for your project because you can easily reach all your supplies. If you create several centers, make a list of the centers and keep it somewhere you can easily notice.

Simple Methods to Maintain a Freshly Organized Space

The Handy Box
When cleaning out a room, have a handy box or basket to gather items that are in inappropriate locations. After cleaning the room, return the items to their proper positions.

In the Moment
- Close an open drawer when you pass by.
- Empty a full waste basket when you pass by.
- Pick up a clothing item lying carelessly on the floor.
- Place loose papers in the to-file box.
- 10-minute pickup.
- Every night, spend ten minutes picking stuff up. Grab a basket and

walk around your house picking misplaced items and returning them to their proper locations. If you live with your family, ask them to clean their spaces in the evening before bedtime.

Speed Clean

- Pick up dropped items.
- Replace whatever you use to its rightful position.
- Clean spills immediately.

Just 15 Minutes

This tactic helps you get started on tasks.

- Start a 15-minute timer.
- Concentrate on your tasks for 15 minutes.
- When the timer goes off, determine if you want to continue for another 15 minutes.
- If you can, set the timer again.
- If you cannot, stop for the moment and try again some other time using the same process until you have completed the task.
- Seeing how much you have accomplished in 15 minutes will surely motivate you.

Subtract Before You Add

Follow the rule of subtraction before adding. This means there will be no addition (buying) of a new item until you have subtracted one. For instance, you can't get a new book unless you have given away unread ones.

Put Things in Place

If you have some spare time, dedicate some of it towards replacing a few items that are not placed correctly. This could be your kids' toys, clothing, or whatever else you can find in your home.

Have a Throw or Donate Box

Keep a bag or box handy to store items for donation. When you notice an item you no longer need, put it inside the donate box. Be careful not to allow unwanted stuff to clog valuable space while waiting for a general clean up day. If the items are too small to donate, trash them.

HOW TO INCREASE PRODUCTIVITY AS AN ADULT WITH ADHD

If you have ADHD, chances are, you have troubles with being productive. How do you remain productive with your disorder? Well, here are some tips that can help you. Practice all the techniques until you discover the best one for you.

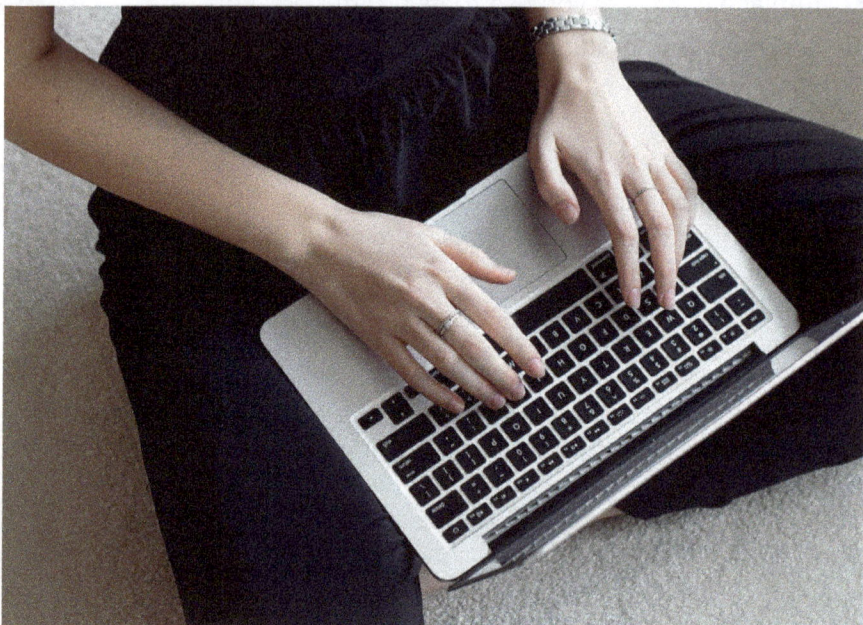

Create a Working Organizational Strategy
Since there is no uniform solution to organizational problems, you have to try all the strategies until you find your match.

The organizational strategies can be
- a journal
- a traditional planner
- calendar (wall or online)
- organizational apps
- whiteboard

When you find the strategy that fits you, practice it for a minimum of 30 days. Go everywhere with it and record every detail about you. With time, you'll get used to it.

Make Your Daily Plans at Night

Rather than being hit with confusion every morning on what tasks to focus on for the day, make your plans the night before. Put your to-do list somewhere it's easy to spot like on your nightstand, clothes closet, or bathroom mirror. Doing this gives you an idea where to start your day.

Start Your Day with an Exciting Task

People with ADHD often fear starting a project or task. In most cases, the thought of doing their task for the day keeps them stagnant. However, you can change that by making the first activity of your day pleasurable. You could choose to start with a delicious breakfast, a chat with a friend, or a favorite exercise routine. Start your day with something that will keep you excited to continue with other tasks.

Build Momentum

Check your to-do list to note the hardest and the easiest tasks. It may help to begin the day with tasks that seem the easiest, create a pattern, and move gradually into hard things. If you can, list the top three priorities on the list and finish with them. When this is done, you are assured that all your important tasks are complete.

Regardless of whether you choose to start with the easy or hard tasks, ensure that you put more energy into tasks that will give you a higher feeling of accomplishment. This gives you the momentum to approach other tasks.

Have an Intention

One of the most common forms of distraction are our mobile devices. Checking our devices during the day for social media and work messages is easy. And we often get lost in it. This happens even to individuals without Attention Deficit Hyperactive Disorder. But it might be more difficult to do certain tasks if you have the condition.

Before you grab your phone, have an intention and decide what you need to do with it and how long it will take. That is, your plan may be to dedicate 10 minutes to social media and 30 minutes on emails. After the allocated time elapses, leave the devices alone and continue with your task.

Work in Intervals

Get a stopwatch and set a timer for 45 minutes. Alternatively, set it on your phone. Within the 45 minutes, throw yourself into your tasks and avoid distraction from any source. After the timer beeps, take a 15 minutes break.

Do this over and over when necessary. If 45 minutes is too long for you, do a 15-minute-on and 5-minute-off interval. As you continue the practice, your concentration level increases.

Don't Multitask

People brag about multitasking a lot. But this can be detrimental to your productivity. Engaging in little side tasks will keep you from concentrating on your main work and getting it done. In the end, you'll probably have lots of unfinished projects. Concentrate on one task at once.

Remove Distractions

Work in a quiet place and ensure your phone is on silent mode. If necessary, disable your social media notifications while you work. After work, you can turn on your notifications again.

Carve Out a Work Zone

If you work from home, create a work center away from the place you eat, sleep, or have fun.

Set up your workstation in a quiet place where there is less clutter and physical distractions. If you have a window that opens to a natural view, set your work station there. Let your mind associate your work zone with business. Your mind can switch away when you leave the work station.

Pace Yourself

Perfection is usually the goal of most people with ADHD. You might refuse to start a project entirely because you can't be perfect.

Approach your project with the mindset of completing your requirements first. After accomplishing that, you can decide to put in extra touches to the project. Don't bother about the finishing until you have started from the foundation.

Pair Up With an Accountability Partner

Most times we don't realize our deadlines are close until they are staring us right in the face. You might keep your task pending until the last minute causing more problems with the project. Get an accountability partner to keep you from putting your tasks off until the deadline.

Impose a deadline on yourself that is different from your official one. Have your accountability partner know that you are presenting a certain part of your project by a certain date. Send the work to them after it is completed. Knowing that you have someone waiting to receive your work will drive you to concentrate.

Have a Buffer

Being productive with ADHD takes time. Cut yourself some slack, especially if you are yet to build a proper productivity routine. If you have to do a project in 3 hours, map out 6 hours in your schedule as a safety net. You'll be better off overestimating than underestimating.

Build a Brain Dump

Usually, your mind gets distracted if you need to finish an urgent task. Have a brain dump, which is a small notebook where you can record everything your mind comes up with during work. When you get the thought off your head, it no longer bothers you.

CHAPTER 4

ADHD AND MEMORY

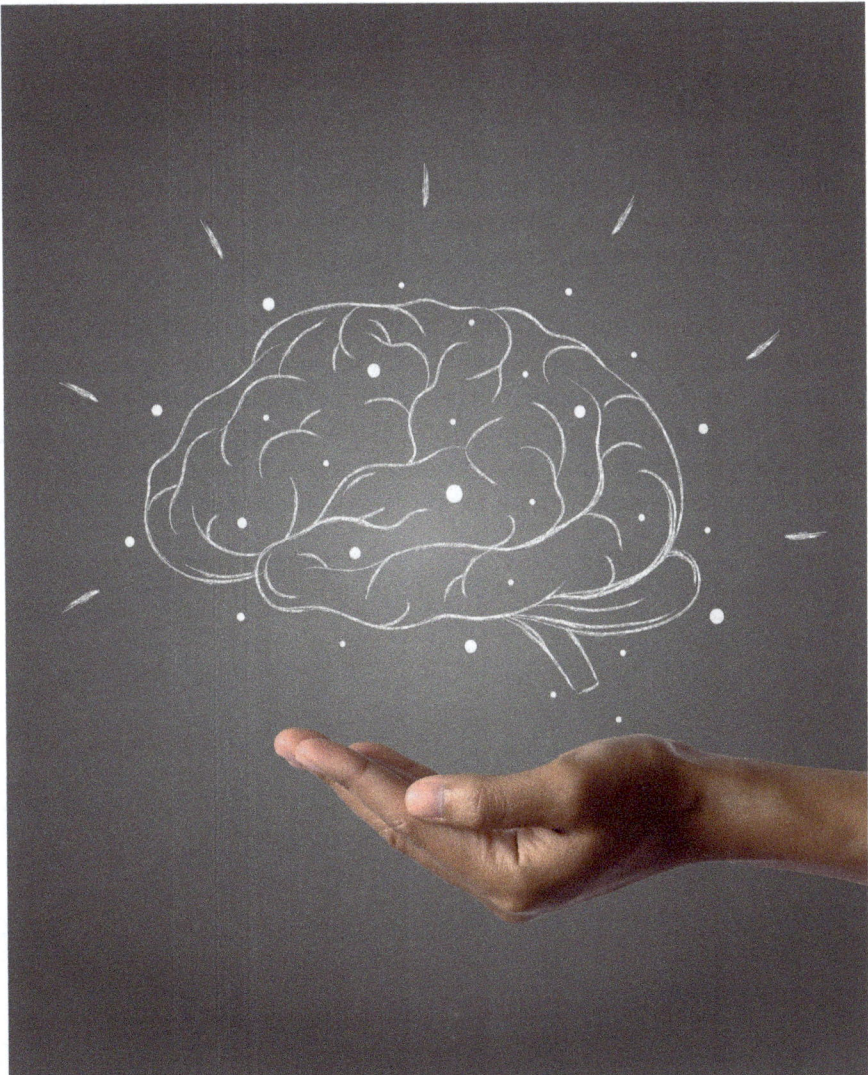

People with ADHD struggle with several memory problems, like short-term and long-term memory. Common ADHD symptoms like inattentiveness affects the storage and coding of information in the memory. Since most adults with ADHD are not as attentive to their environment as they should be, they seldom build memories of information.

CONNECTING ADHD TO WORKING MEMORY

The working memory is the short term storage system in the brain where many thoughts are held as the individual performs a task. The presence of a working memory in the brain is for individuals to store information for a while until it is needed and they can move on to the next item. It is the part of the memory that supports daily achievements, like organizing tasks, following guidelines, making plans, and following a schedule. Think about working on a paper and having different sources open on several tabs.

It is your working memory that helps you recall the information in the different tabs, the one you have just read, and the way you want to structure the paragraph you have currently. The scenario where you enter a room and forget why you're there (which happens to most people anyway) is known as a "memory lapse." People with ADHD have frequent memory lapses than those who do not.

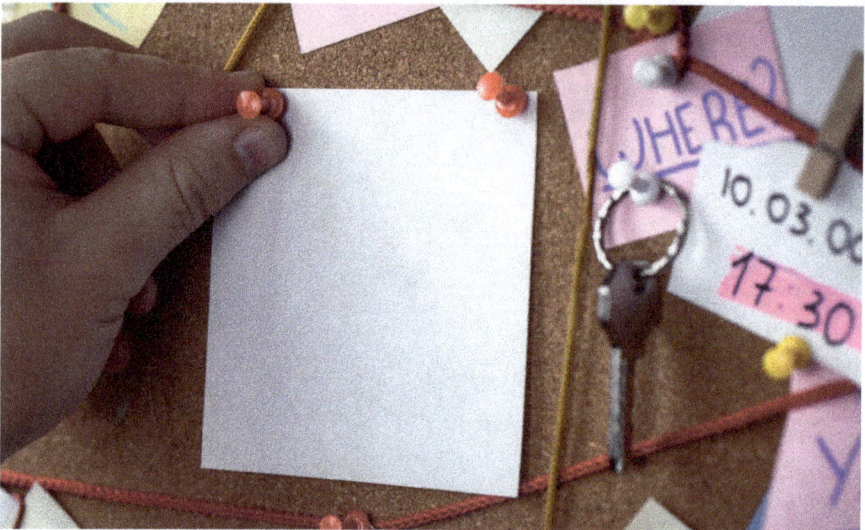

These are ways in which your life is affected by ADHD:

- You decide to say your opinion in a conversation, but you forget what you had in mind once it's your turn to talk.
- You regularly misplace your cell phone, wallet, or keys.
- You are easily lost even after receiving directions.
- You have difficulty sticking to conversations because you keep forgetting what the others say.
- You have a backlog of unfinished projects because you're easily distracted and forget what you're working on.
- You make plans to finish tasks at home but forget to come along with necessary tools.
- You need to read a paragraph over and over before the information sticks.
- You frequently miss deadlines because you're disorganized and lack the capacity to complete projects.

ADHD and Long-term Memory

The long term memory is not exempted from the effects of ADHD. People with ADHD often perform poorly on long-term memory tests. Experts suggest that the memory problems of ADHD are more related to memory encoding than retrieval. This is because the individual with ADHD barely forms memories, and so they cannot retrieve much information. With all the memory problems that people with ADHD struggle with, others often expect them to have problems with intelligence.

People with ADHD usually do not have low IQ. Even with the cognitive problems they might suffer, their intelligence level is around average or above average. They prefer to learn at their own pace and their bad grades at school were often because they were expected to do tasks they are unmotivated for.

Improving Working Memory

Everyone can improve their working memory. The working memory can be easily trained with exercise because of its flexibility.

You can fix your working memory problems using several exercises. For example, there are many working memory challenges online which can test your recollection skills and enhance your working memory. The downside, however, is that these benefits may be temporary and fade off after the training.

But research shows that committing to a brain training may lead to major improvements (Godman, 2014). If you want to improve your working memory, you should first understand the way memory works and accept your limits.

These are some helpful strategies to improve working memory:

1. **Divide complex information into simpler chunks:** When you receive information that feels overwhelming, break it down. Work on one or two problems before you move on to another. For instance, if you have to throw a party in your home, the process of getting things in order may be overwhelming. You need to shop, clean, cook, and set up the area. Concentrate on one aspect, like cleaning. Don't pay attention to the other tasks until you are done with cleaning.

2. **Make a checklist if the task has multiple procedures:** Create a checklist to micromanage your activities. For instance, you can choose to make one for your first hour at work. In the checklist you may add returning calls, listening to messages, replying emails, checking yesterday's update, meeting with supervisor to complete important tasks, etc.

3. **Start routines:** The importance of routines for people with ADHD cannot be overemphasized. They help you have a grip on your activities. Having a routine can be as little as dropping your keys in the same spot every time you return home.

4. **Practice working memory skills:** Register for online brain training programs. Alternatively, you can make your own. Jot down six unrelated words. Try to remember the first two words you've written without stealing a glance. If you succeed, write another word.

5. **Try different means of remembering information:** People recall lists easily when they turn it into a song or a rhyme. You can practice that. You can also try recalling multiple items by visualizing them. For instance, you need to pick up some items from the store. While you head home from work, picture yourself stopping at the store and gathering each of the supplies you need. Imagine yourself at the different sections of the store. Because imagery is more powerful than words, your visualization will help you recall the items that you need.

6. **Avoid multitasking:** Multitasking is not exactly as great as people say it is. It could possibly shrink different areas of your brain as it has a relationship to short attention spans. Focus on one task at a time. If this is too much of a struggle, set alarms to capture all your attention on a single task within a short period. This reduces distraction from multiple side tasks and keeps you from forgetting your main task.

7. **Practice mindfulness:** Mindfulness can also help you focus and boost working memory. A daily practice can increase your ability to recall and helps you learn to regulate sensory input and tune out distractions.

8. **Exercise daily:** Daily exercise has been shown to have a positive effect on the working memory. Physical activity can boost brain health and further improve your cognitive abilities including working memory.

9. **Use your medication:** The stimulant medications prescribed for people with ADHD can improve the brain areas that are linked to working memory.

10. **Attend therapy:** Therapy can help reduce ADHD linked memory problems. With treatments like cognitive behavioral therapy, you can learn to change your thought patterns and behavior. Learning new coping skills can help with your memory.

11. **Embrace technology:** If you have problems with your memory, learn to program your day with apps and smart devices. You can find apps or programs designed for people with ADHD to boost your concentration.

→ If you want something simple, create reminders in your phone's calendar for the activities that you have. If you're worried about missing an appointment, schedule a reminder as soon as you book the appointment for up to 1 day, 1 hour, or 30 minutes before the time.

12. **Practice positive self-talk:** Everyone talks to themselves sometimes. Self-talk is a great way to organize your thoughts. However, it can be harmful to your productivity if you are too critical of yourself. Be positive during your self-talk and shower yourself with encouragement and love. Don't punish yourself for your mistakes, but rather maintain positivity and optimism to work through it.

→ If you continually struggle with focusing on a task, rather than berating yourself with statements like, "You're such a failure," and, "You can't concentrate on the simplest tasks," say things like, "I have worked so hard on this task for so long. I should take a quick break and return to do better at it."

13. **Ask others for help:** This depends on how comfortable you are with those around you. Ask your close pals to help you remember things. Let them know the reason for asking and the kind of reminders you'll appreciate.

→ Ask people in your home to remind you of chores you need to do. Delegate friends to send you reminders of birthdays and anniversaries within your circle. You might also want to ask your neighbors to send reminders for you to wheel out your trash or ask a colleague to text you when it's time to start preparing for a meeting.

BRAIN EXERCISES TO REFORM WORKING MEMORY

Many of the online games recommended to build memory do not always work. Most times the effects are temporary. The apps only train you to complete memory tasks within the app world. The strategies are not applicable to the real word, hence the effects disappear once you get off the online space. The kind of memory exercises you need are practical exercises that boost your ability to make connections or improve your focus.

Basically, the best brain fitness exercise for a person with ADHD should not only provide abstract training, but real life application and usage. Any brain fitness exercise has to be channeled towards specific goals in order to achieve substantial outcome and prevent further decline of the cognitive abilities.

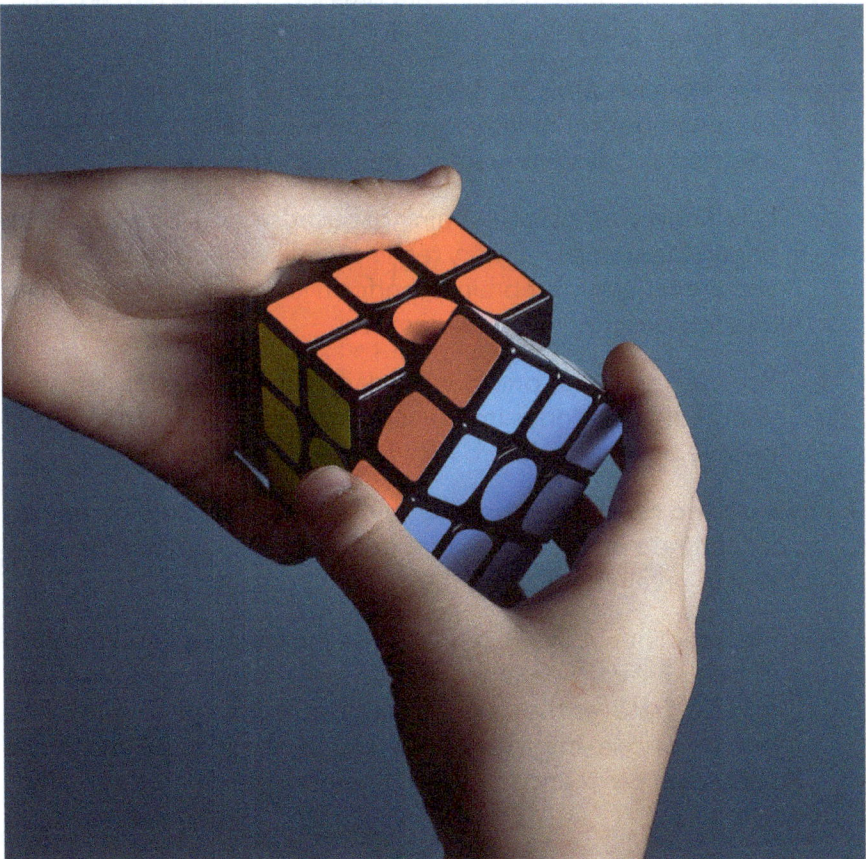

These are some practical exercises that can help you train your brain:

1. **Number brain exercises to enhance concentration:** Numeracy is one way to enhance your cognitive abilities as they facilitate improvement in your logical thinking. You could practice with this brain workout: "Add 3 minus 7." To play this, you need to pick any 3 digit number and do an addition of 3 to your choice digits three different times. Subtract 7 from the final digit 7 times.

   → Do this over and over; about 5 times. Each time you try, choose a new 3 digit number. You can also decide to start with different numbers of variables, like a 4 digit number.

2. **The 4 detail observation exercise:** In this case, you will have to stretch your observation skills. When you meet people in public, try to notice four details about them. For instance, when you meet someone, note that they are dressed in a blue hat, red shirt, brown shoes, and have brown hair.

   → This exercise aims to have you observe the details and try to remember them later. Some scientists refer to this kind of exercise as "passive memory training."

   → It is known as passive training because you don't have to engage in special memory techniques like mnemonics. Rather, you are tasking your brain to perform its original programming and job description: to remember.

   → You can start with one person daily. If you are confident that your memorization is improving, then increase the number of people or information to recall.

3. **Repeat and recall what people say:** Your brain should be trained to concentrate on the things that people in your environment say and try to recall them later.

   → First, register your presence in the moment by keeping track of peoples' conversations with you by repeating them in your mind. Whatever they say, repeat it quietly in your mind. This brain exercise improves your cognitive function and helps your short-term and long-term memory to remember more.

4. **Metronome clapping exercise:** Put on a metronome at slow speed and try to "cover the click." This neurobic exercise teaches your brain to concentrate on things it can be automated to do. It helps you focus more on your surroundings and improves your memory skills.

5. **Visualization exercises:** You can boost your memory by visualizing several things. It could be events, locations, conversations, etc. All you have to do is create pictures in your head. For instance, you can conjure images of your favorite actor in a movie or your favorite artist on stage. Conjuring random images can be incredibly helpful to you. The ideas and images you create will be part of a mnemonics dictionary that lives in you.

6. **Create a memory palace:** One of the best ways to boost brain function also doubles as the easiest. It's simply a drawing but with some accompanying principles.

   → The process of making a memory palace is connected to your spatial and visual memory. It also exercises the recovered memory and autobiographical memory. Unlike other mind exercises, the memory palace training exercise has a reverse approach. This is due to the fact that you are triggered to draw upon visual memory cues that are locked in your mind away from your awareness.

   → Here's how it goes: You probably never go into a new home or store with the conscious decision of memorizing it. But when you recall the home of the last friend you visited, you are able to remember an incredible amount of details. This might be quite difficult for you with ADHD, but the memory palace helps you flex that innate ability. It can work for you to learn other things too.

   → Creating a memory tool is a lifetime tool. The moment you create and master how to use one, you are able to create more and more of them. And when you can, your memory allows you to do extraordinary things. For instance, you become skilled at recalling names at events or reaching your memory goals.

7. **Learn a foreign language:** Being multilingual is a great way to improve the brain. This is chiefly because you're always tasking your brain to recall something. Learning a new language utilizes your brain's neuroplasticity. People of different ages can practice this exercise because it sharpens the brain's ability to learn new things, while also providing the opportunity to relate with more people.

→ With regular conversation, your mind will be stimulated to trigger the release of healthy chemicals which improves mental health. Learning a new language ideally involves using study materials and books. Having conversations about those things pokes at different levels of your memory, especially verbal memory.

→ If talking is a chore for you, singing is also just as effective. You can do either or both. Researchers have discovered that singing decreases cortisol levels and triggers other healing chemicals (Sublet, 2020). If you are singing in a foreign language, the effect on your brain is heightened. As with learning any other new activity, learning a new language triggers the formation of new neural pathways making you boost brain power.

8. **Mind mapping for maximum brain health:** Mind mapping means brainstorming and planning, but visually. It works for when you need to take notes and review. Mind mapping is effective at improving cognitive function because it reproduces the role of nerve cells on paper.

→ For instance, the same way a brain cell has a main nucleus with synapses that branch out, the mind map has a main idea which supplies mental power to other idea streams. When you create mind maps, you reduce the pressure on your brain, leaving it free to handle other stuff. Therefore increasing its processing speed.

9. **Sports and fitness as a memory exercise:** Exercise is great. In addition to keeping your muscles toned and your heart rate up, physical activity is an awesome technique for a mental workout.

→ For instance, memorizing the number of sets and reps you do is a great memory exercise. During or after your tai chi session, you can practice recalling your memory palaces. Also, rather than watching TV while running on the treadmill, you can try recalling and practicing some words in the foreign language you're learning.

→ When you get on the stationary bike, or during your high intensity interval breaks, you can do the four detail exercise while watching people. Physical exercise, in addition to boosting your memory, helps relieve stress and reduce the symptoms of ADHD.

CHAPTER 5

ADHD: OVERCOMING THE SHAME

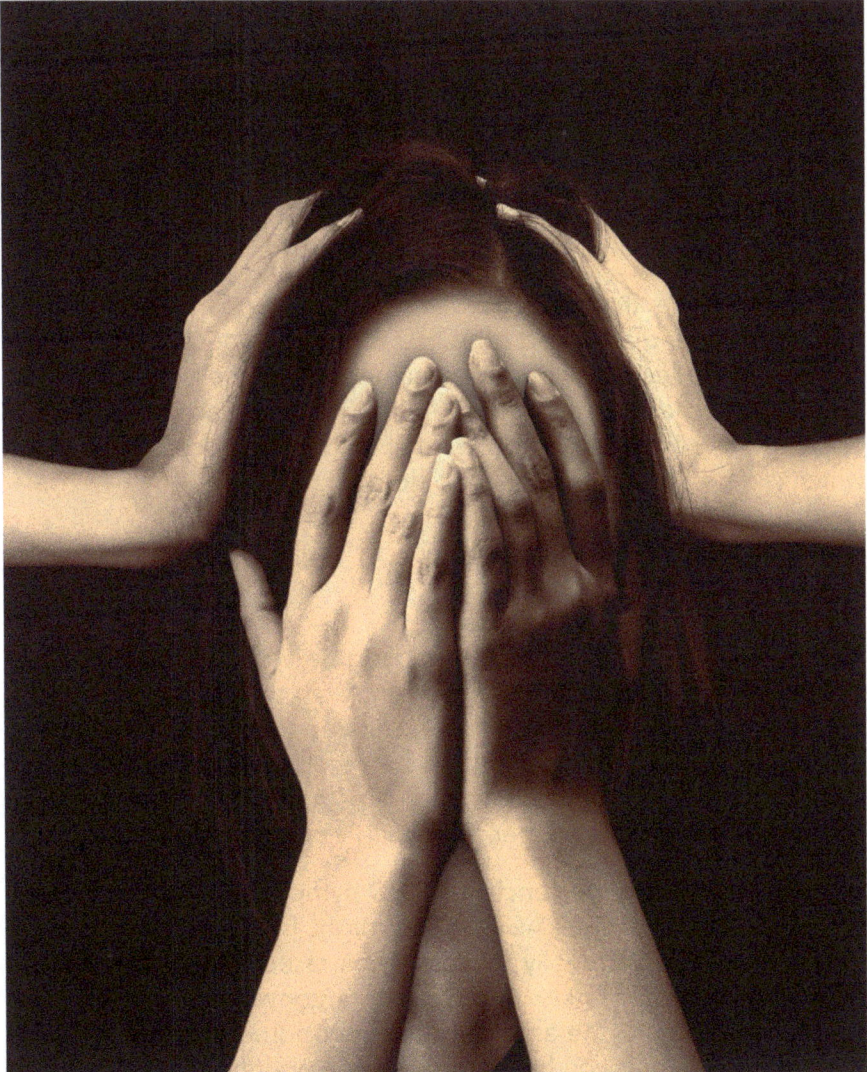

As a person with ADHD, it might be incredibly difficult to manage all your symptoms. Your best efforts may not be enough to reach people's expectations, making you feel like you are letting everyone down. Having this feeling can result in shame.

Despite how difficult your symptoms are, you should never be ashamed of ADHD. As you work on your symptoms and learn coping strategies, you will develop confidence in being a person with ADHD. Shame stems from the belief that your attitude is generally unacceptable in society and different from the norm.

If you have ADHD, you will often behave in ways that upset social norms. For instance, the reactions of people around you when you frequently interrupt a conversation due to brain impulses can trigger shame. The shame of your ADHD may make you respond a certain way even though you know you are not exactly in control of your actions.

You can reduce the feelings of shame if you can reshape your thoughts. Feeling ashamed of ADHD is not ideal because it is a part of you. It implies that you are ashamed of yourself. Trying to put up a different identity from your ADHD persona can be lonely and draining. This is because you will fail to get the necessary support which can help address your condition.

Much of the shame that people with ADHD feel comes in the following ways:

- **Shame about being different:** People with ADHD often feel ashamed because they are different from their friends. This kind of shame is more pronounced in children than adults. It is natural for children to want to blend in with their friends and this makes them aware of things that separate them. And this shame of being different may linger from childhood to adulthood.

- **Shame about experiencing ADHD symptoms:** There are many behavioral effects of ADHD. You might find yourself acting on impulse and eventually feeling embarrased about your actions or having troubles keeping up with a conversation and feeling 'dumb.' You may be ashamed that your home or office is always cluttered or that you have trouble remembering things.

- **Shame about their history:** Do the thoughts of your past records fill you with shame? Do you think about the relationship that didn't work, or the time your forgetfulness made you run out of gas on the highway? You will always feel shame every time your mind returns to embarrassing memories.

- **Shame about their current position:** Many adults with ADHD do not like the point where they are right now in life. Many believe they are failures for not reaching many of the milestones they think they would at their age. Do you feel shame when you see your friends smashing goals that you desire but haven't yet achieved, even though you are as smart and qualified as they are?

HOW A PERSON WITH ADHD DEVELOPS SHAME

Shame begins differently for everyone. If you are ashamed that you have ADHD, it is probably because you have internalised shame partly due to how the people around you (family and teachers) treated you during childhood for being talkative or late. And as you approached adulthood, your friends, partner, colleagues ,and other adults continued to shame you for the same problems.

With time, the criticisms may become your truths. You might accept that you are who they say you are and start to see yourself as a failure who can't get things right.

Regardless of how your shame must have developed, it eventually becomes a hindrance to you.

HOW SHAME HINDERS THE SUCCESS OF YOUR ADHD MANAGEMENT

Besides making you feel awful about yourself, shame can make it difficult for you to embrace strategies that can be effective for managing your ADHD.

Do a little introspection and consider the times you have made statements like

- "When I ask someone to be my accountability partner so I can complete my work, I feel like a child."

- "I should not need to jot down every tiny detail. I should be able to remember it. I'm not dumb!"

- "I am a grown adult anyway. I should be able to do these things on my own."

All of these statements and similar ones stem from the shame that you feel. You cannot make progress on relieving your ADHD symptoms if you do not make attempts to overcome the feelings of shame.

HOW TO OVERCOME SHAME

You can stop the feelings of shame from keeping you back from achieving your goals of having a better life. But first, you need to acknowledge your shame. Then you can work through it. You can discover when and how your shame starts by detecting which part of your body it is felt in.

Take note of the messages and expectations that make you feel ashamed. It could be because people reprimand you for being talkative or for processing information slowly, and many other triggers you might have.

Also, fact check the messages and expectations that make you ashamed. For instance, if you are being berated for not operating like your colleagues, take a step back and think: How realistic is it for you to behave in the same manner as your colleagues? Do you desire to behave like them?

Consider your memory troubles. Are you being reasonable by expecting your to-do list to stay in your head? Decide if the expectations fueling your shame are even realistic.

The tips below will help you effectively deal with the shame that's brought on by ADHD:

- **Talk about it:** Share your ADHD story with others. Your shame may compound when you keep the condition a secret. Talk about ADHD and you will find relief.

- **Confide in someone:** Even if you may be uncomfortable about your shame, it is great to share it with your loved ones. You might be worried that their invalidation may worsen the shame. However, if you can tell your thoughts and feelings to a trusted person, it helps you find an outlet to vent. Sharing with someone can also help you feel less lonely and isolated.

- **Join an ADHD support group:** If you struggle with shame of ADHD, you will get more help when you find people with shared experiences. Organizations like Children and Adults with ADHD (CHADD) provide support groups for people. ADHD coaching can be effective for managing your symptoms and the consequences, including the negative feelings that result like shame.

- **Self-compassion is important:** Because of the shame, you may feel unworthy of being human. However, it's best for you to accept yourself, as ADHD is a scientifically acknowledged disorder. Although ADHD symptoms cause you to express socially unacceptable behavior, it doesn't make you unacceptable as a person.

  → Understanding the difference between you and your disorder will help you be compassionate about yourself so that you can fight the shame.

  → Challenge yourself to figure out the negative thoughts you have about ADHD and determine which of them makes you ashamed. The more understanding you have about those feelings, the better your chances of targeting the perceptions.

- **Discover your triggers:** Have you stopped to find out what triggers your shame? You can take note of a particular experience, location, or person that is making you feel ashamed and mark it as a potential trigger. If you notice the feelings of shame occur very frequently, you should take time to discover what causes you to feel shame all the time.

  → When you know your triggers, you can then search for the main reason why they make you ashamed. For instance, if interrupting a person during conversation makes you ashamed, work on improving active listening and joining the conversation only at appropriate times.

→ You can only find a solution to a trigger if you are able to identify it. For example, if coming in late for meetings makes you ashamed, you can ask a friend to help you with timekeeping, or ask your workplace to make concessions for you. Your feelings of shame may also reduce if you hang around loved ones who understand your struggles.

- **Notice the positives:** Positive feedback will help you overcome shame due to the fact that it gives you a different viewpoint from the negative criticism you have experienced.

  → When you get positive feedback, it serves as a reminder of the improvements going on in your life. You will feel good about yourself and know that you deserve respect with each piece of positive feedback that you get.

  → Monitor all your achievements even if they seem little. Doing this helps you stay on top of your progress. Ensure that you take proper note of all your positives, as they can help you overcome the effects of any other negative feedback you might get.

  → If you have been feeling ashamed of ADHD, you might want to discuss your situation with a therapist. A qualified mental health professional will help you work through strategies to combat challenging situations. An ADHD specialist will help you figure out different ways to manage your shame and eventually reduce it.

ADHD MYTHS AND FACTS

Over the years, there's been a lot of misconception about ADHD. People have spread different opinions about ADHD, and has resulted in some confusion about the true nature of the disorder. To address your disorder, you should be able to identify the myths being propagated and counter them with real facts. Below are some of the myths of ADHD that have been debunked.

ADHD Is Not a Real Medical Condition

Many people are convinced that ADHD is merely a made-up condition.

Fact: ADHD has gained recognition as a medical condition from the National Institutes of Health, the Centers for Disease Control and Prevention, and the American Psychiatric Association. It is a very common childhood disorder. The US records millions of kids and adults with ADHD. Imaging studies have detected that the brain development of people with ADHD is different from those who do not have the disorder. If you live with ADHD, you understand the reality and the extent of its impact on daily life.

People With ADHD Just Need to Try Harder

Most people believe that ADHD people are just not making enough effort to deal with their symptoms.

Fact: ADHD is not a consequence of demotivation. People who have it are always doing the best they can to pay attention. Saying people with ADHD "just need to focus" is the same as asking a myopic person to see farther. Their attention problems are not in any way connected to their attitude. Their brain functions are just wired and structured in a different way.

People With ADHD Can Never Concentrate

Everyone knows people with ADHD have difficulty focusing or concentrating. However, most people believe they will never achieve focus or concentrate on a task.

Fact: Granted, people with ADHD struggle with concentrating. However, when they develop an interest in something, they channel intense focus on it. This situation is known as 'hyperfocus.' Basically, they go overboard when focusing on things they are genuinely interested in. This is why some children with ADHD may be easily distracted in class but have a harder time detaching themselves from playtime. Adults may face difficulty working on boring projects, but put in all their best into parts of the job that they like.

Every Child With ADHD Is Hyperactive

People picture a child with ADHD as the restless kid running all over the place. But there is more to this.

Fact: While the ADHD stereotype is a child who never stops moving, that is untrue for all cases. The hyperactivity symptom is not present in all children and when it does, it goes away or reduces as the child grows. As mentioned in earlier chapters of the book, ADHD presents in three types. The Inattention type of ADHD does not affect the activity levels of the individual.

ADHD Only Occurs In Boys

People assume only boys have ADHD. This stems from the myth that the symptoms are only limited to hyperactivity.

Fact: The ratio of diagnosis of ADHD in boys and girls is 2:1. This proves that girls do have it. Often, the symptoms they experience are overlooked and the disorder remains undetected. This is partly because ADHD manifests differently in boys and girls. Girls do not often struggle with hyperactivity or impulsivity as much as boys. The symptoms make them appear more 'daydreamy' than restless.

ADHD Is a Learning Disability

Because ADHD affects cognitive abilities, people are quick to brand it a learning disability.

Fact: ADHD is not a learning disability. True, the symptoms can affect learning negatively, but there is no effect on particular skills like writing, math, and reading. ADHD, however, can coexist with certain learning disabilities. This coexistence partly fuels the myth. Regardless of its status as a learning disability, children with ADHD can still get help in school, while adults with ADHD can be provided with support at work.

Children With ADHD Outgrow It

People commonly associate ADHD with the hyperactivity of children. Hence, they see it as a condition that only affects children, which they'll eventually outgrow.

Fact: Many children do not outgrow ADHD completely, even though some of the symptoms can reduce or disappear with time. The symptoms might change when the child grows and figures out strategies to manage them. However, that's a lot different from outgrowing it. Many individuals with ADHD still have symptoms even as adults.

ADHD Is Caused by Poor Parenting

This myth is often fueled by the hyperactive symptoms of ADHD. People assume that the children are badly behaved, and so it has to be their parent's fault.

Fact: ADHD results from changes in the structure of the brain—not bad parenting. People often believe children with ADHD that fidget or act on impulse are just not disciplined. Many don't understand that it is a medical condition way beyond the action or inaction of parents or caregivers.

Medication Is the Only Treatment Method

Since it is described as a medical condition, people believe it can only be treated by medicines.

Fact: People should understand that ADHD cannot be cured. The treatment options available only serve to manage the symptoms.

Medication is one of the many treatment options. Medications for ADHD include stimulants and non-stimulants. These two classes of medicines provide some relief for people with ADHD. People react differently to medication and so the physician may need to administer several types of medications until they find the most suitable.

Behavioral therapy is the second treatment option, which helps the individual rechannel their thoughts and shut out distractions. Many physicians recommend a combination of medication and therapy to effectively manage the symptom.

People With ADHD Are Lazy

People who don't understand ADHD often refer to people with the disorder as lazy.

Fact: Many people with ADHD receive accusations of being lazy, and this causes them to feel guilty for their low productivity and motivation. Individuals with ADHD require extra structure, reminders, and concessions to go through activities that need continuous mental effort. However, some symptoms of ADHD, which include disorganization, lack of interest, and motivation (except in activities that they genuinely enjoy), are erroneously thought to be laziness.

A person with ADHD may see sorting through an email to be as demanding as writing a class exam. But normal people see these tasks as simple and therefore wrongfully conclude that the person with ADHD is lazy.

This myth may cause people with ADHD to develop self-esteem issues due to negative feelings that arise from not completing supposedly simple tasks.

ADHD Is Not That Serious

Fact: ADHD is not fatal, but it seriously affects the general quality of a person's life. People with ADHD have higher chances of developing anxiety and mood disorders, abusing substances, and many others.

Many people with ADHD have trouble meeting work demands and are regularly monitored and placed on probation. They are in constant fear of being fired from their jobs and being financially unstable. Eventually, this fear affects their personal life. People with ADHD need more time to finish tasks and may find support in educational settings. But the workforce may not accommodate their struggles, hence the frequent loss of jobs.

CHAPTER 6

CHALLENGES THAT PEOPLE WITH ADHD FACE

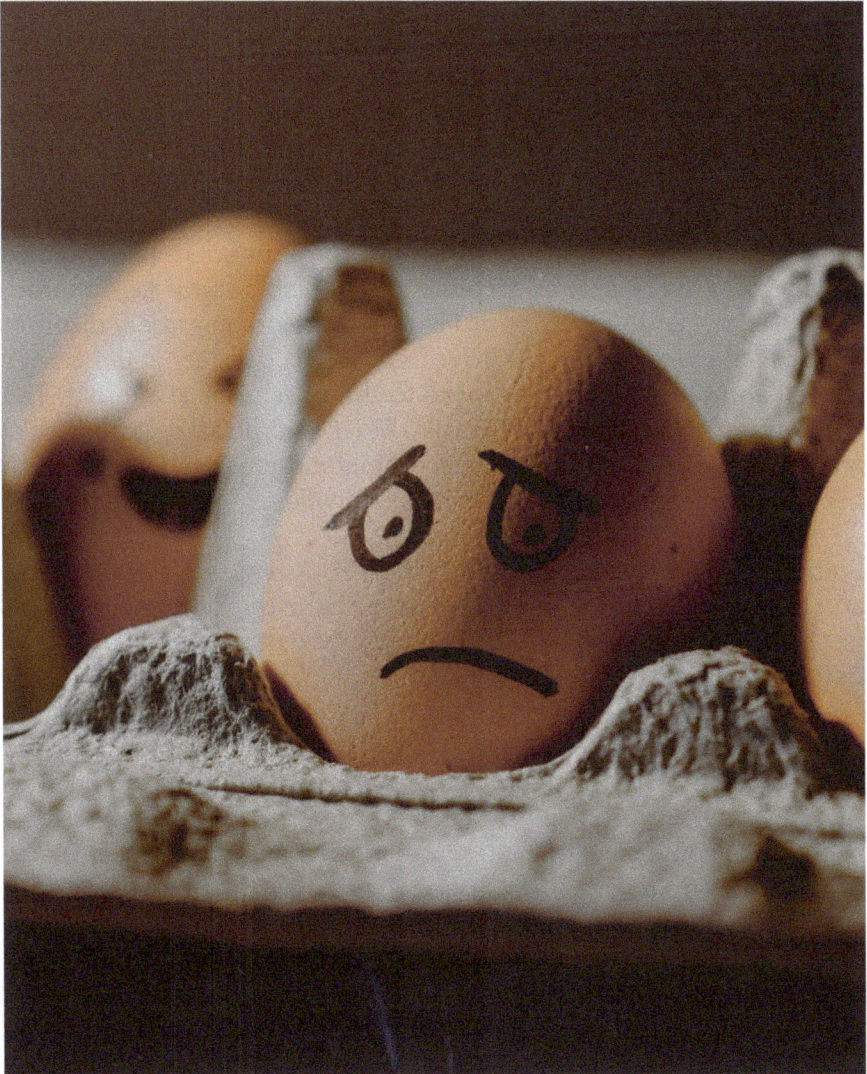

In previous chapters, some of the challenges of people with ADHD were mentioned. However, this chapter seeks to elucidate and provide clarity to them.

ADHD AND ANXIETY

People with ADHD lead anxious lives. Because of the nature of the disorder, ordinary daily activities are stressful for them. There's always an element of uncertainty in every environment and situation they find themselves in. As a result, it is very necessary to discuss ADHD and its relationship to anxiety. People with ADHD may either worry frequently about certain things or activities, like work deadlines or school work, or struggle with actual anxiety disorders. Nonetheless, ADHD has a direct relationship with anxiety, and the latter is the most common mental health problem to coexist with adult ADHD.

While anxiety is not one of the symptoms needed to diagnose ADHD, they have a strong connection which cannot be ignored. People with ADHD are twice as likely to develop an anxiety disorder than people without the disorder (Issa, 2021). Anxiety is the body's mental and physiological response to the possibility of a threat. The different kinds of anxiety disorder, like panic attacks, ptsd, social anxiety disorder, and others, cause debilitating fear and worry which negatively affects an individual's daily activities.

Some symptoms which people with ADHD present, like fidgeting and trouble with concentration, are also characteristic of anxiety. This necessitates physicians to rule out anxiety and other mental disorders before an ADHD diagnosis is confirmed, and vice versa.

People whose anxiety disorders coexist with ADHD present more severe anxiety symptoms than those without ADHD. Still, adults with ADHD who do not qualify to receive an anxiety disorder diagnosis experience some level of anxiety in their everyday lives just because of ADHD. People with ADHD often lose track of time, have a poor working memory, experience intense emotions, and other anxiety-based symptoms. When people with ADHD are anxious in any situation, their ADHD symptoms become worse. This happens when there is some level of uncertainty about the outcome of an event or task.

"Consistent inconsistency" accurately describes the experience of anxiety for a person with ADHD. It depicts the distrust and uncertainty that a person with ADHD develops after many years of struggling with ADHD symptoms. If you have ADHD, you might experience anxiety and be totally unsure of everything around you. The concept of "consistent inconsistency" explains the situation where you are aware of the need to complete a task but you are unsure of your ability to do so.

ADHD = performance anxiety (in most cases).

People with ADHD know what needs to be done, and in most cases, know how to do it. Still, they struggle with implementation, which makes them stressed and eventually fuels anxiety. This is why ADHD in adults is overwhelming.

The following cause struggle with implementation:

- **Self regulatory efficacy:** In this case, the person admits their ability to handle a task, as well as uncertainty of the ability to complete it. The mindset goes, "I am sure I can do this, but I am not sure I can concentrate or avoid distraction."

- **Incautious optimism:** In this case, the person has twisted positivity. They usually think, "I am more productive at the last minute."

- **Front end perfectionism:** Adults with ADHD often have extremely high standards and say things like, "I need to be in the mood / have plenty of energy to take action."

- **Emotional dysregulation:** Although the DSM-5 does not include this as a symptom, intense emotions are a major feature of ADHD. Part of controlling nervousness is having the option to change and regulate our emotional states so we can promptly participate in an assignment. If the individual cannot adequately handle discomfort, they tend to avoid and procrastinate, and this triggers and can be triggered by anxiety.

THE DISTINCTION BETWEEN ADHD AND ANXIETY

While these two conditions may share some symptoms, they are entirely different. Anxiety is majorly a disorder characterized by excessive worry, fear, and nervousness, while ADHD is a disorder marked by inattentiveness. Individuals with anxiety present certain compulsive or perfectionist behaviors that do not accompany ADHD symptoms.

The difference between the two conditions lie in the frequency and the situation that triggers the experience. While a person with anxiety disorder may not concentrate in some conditions that make them anxious, one with ADHD lacks concentration most or all of the time. Even though the symptoms of both conditions may seem quite obvious, proper evaluation and diagnosis need to be made before a conclusion.

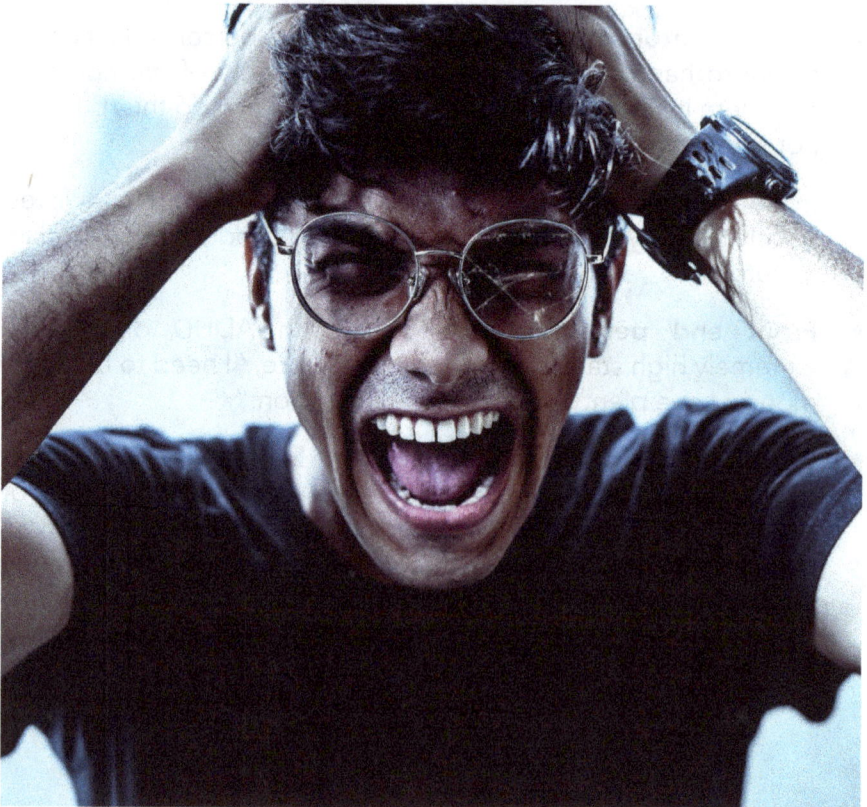

HOW TO TREAT BOTH ADHD AND ANXIETY

Medication and psychotherapy are the choice treatments for ADHD and anxiety. Most times treating only one of the conditions improves the symptoms of both in some individuals. If the two conditions coexist, physicians often choose to treat the one with the most severe symptoms.

The stimulant medications provided for people with ADHD do not exacerbate anxiety symptoms, and non-stimulants are regarded as the next best choice for treating coexisting ADHD and anxiety. Most people find more relief from a combination of medication and therapy. People with ADHD who also struggle with anxiety can get better by developing healthy coping strategies.

MANAGING EMOTIONS, BEHAVIOR, AND MINDSET

Understanding your feelings and emotions is the best foundation for learning how to manage your emotions. The onset of anxiety or other confusing feelings can trigger you to ask, "What is this distress signalling?" You may even probe further by asking yourself the following questions:

- What exactly do I feel?
- What is the problem?
- What triggered it?
- Is there any need to worry about this problem? If so, how will it be managed?
- What is the best, worst, and most likely outcome of this problem?

To manage these issues, try the following.

Make Notes

You can choose to write the details of the problem on your phone or computer, but writing with a pen on paper can be a more therapeutic way to air out your worries and stressors. Whichever way you choose to go about it is fine. The most important thing is getting the problem out of your head and seeing it as text. This way you can better understand which part of your problem is in your control and which part is not. Doing this exercise helps you challenge the problem head on.

Here's a look at a practical example of this exercise. What will you do if, for instance, you notice you are self-medicating through alcohol? These steps might help: Ask, "What do I feel," "How does this behavior benefit me," and, "What's in it for me?" Behaviors like this are often linked to the desire to reduce anxiety, prevent stress, and regain control. Acknowledge the situation going on by labeling your feelings. You could be anxious, overwhelmed, or feeling out of control. Knowing exactly what you're feeling can help you relax.

Figure Out Your Triggers

You probably gave in to anxiety due to some degree of personal trauma. The most common ones, however, are loneliness, boredom, stress from work, home troubles, or social obligations.

Carefully Consider These Problems and Triggers

Think hard about the supposed problems. Are they relevant? Have you considered the fact that you're stressing over a particular task because you've given yourself an unrealistic deadline? Have you thought about the best and worst case scenarios? What is the most realistic outcome? When you carefully think about the problem, you may detect a pattern of stressing over things that should ordinarily not be an issue for you.

Find Ways to Handle the Problem

In this scenario, self-medicating on alcohol is a problem that needs fixing. You could either choose to control the stimulus by getting rid of temptations around you, or towing the path of replacement behaviors where you replace alcohol with other liquids or stimuli. Consider seeing a mental health physician if you cannot manage the problem on your own.

COPING STRATEGIES FOR ADHD AND ANXIETY

The tips below will help you live a less worry and anxiety filled life:

- **Create a routine:** You need a clear routine if you want to manage your ADHD and anxiety. The routine you create must also be visible. You can use a calendar on the wall, a digital planner, or an appointment planner. Use the planners to structure the time you have for your daily activities. Be sure to include periods for breaks.

- **Exercise and movement:** Find time in your schedule to exercise. Apart from exercise, regular movements like taking a short walk to the parking lot, or somewhere really close, can do wonders for you. Try as much as you can to move regularly especially if you work from home. Movement and exercise helps you reset.

- **Develop healthy habits:** Even people without ADHD deal with chronic stress, and are usually overwhelmed with one aspect of their life. With ADHD, it could be worse. Maintaining a healthy lifestyle like getting enough sleep, eating an improved diet, and frequent exercise can reduce physical anxiety triggers.

- **Itemize your tasks:** If you have work to do, rather than grouping them all together, break them into different items based on the nature of the tasks or time needed to accomplish it. For instance, rather than inputting "review work report" on your calendar, write, "15 minute or 15 page activity." Checking your emails can be put as "5 emails or 5 minute activity." When you detail the tasks you need to work on, it goes a long way in avoiding front end perfectionism. It helps you work on tasks which you previously didn't have the 'mood' or 'energy' for.

- **Arrange your living space:** If things are clustered around the home, you may need a little more definition. Assign separate corners of your home to work, leisure, and sleep. This way you can form a habit of associating different areas with different activities. Ensure you do not clutter your spaces by preparing them for the next day. This helps you move on quickly into other activities.

- **Continue to use ADHD medication:** Reduce your symptoms by sticking to your prescribed medication(s). If you have started psychotherapy lessons, ensure you continue with them. Treatment measures for ADHD are effective at reducing symptoms, helping you cope and reducing anxiety.

- Decatastrophize: Be grateful for the amount of progress you have made and refuse to dwell on the failures or loss. Even though you expect a certain outcome, try to be flexible with these expectations. Also, see some negative thoughts as plain thoughts which may not have any impact on you.

ADHD AND BOREDOM

As an adult with ADHD, you're no stranger to the feelings of boredom. Whenever you don't feel occupied, you become restless and annoyed so much that it hurts. This feeling triggers you to find something interesting that you can partake in—immediately. If you succeed in finding something that interests you, the feeling of bliss is often unmatched.

Now, think about a scenario where your boredom pushes you to make statements or take actions that you regret later. At that point, it was probably a joke for you, or just something you did to get rid of boredom without caring about the effects on others.

If you cannot recognize these periods of boredom and regulate how you react to it, you may be creating consequences which may create an unpleasant picture of you and your actions.

Therefore, when you think about managing your ADHD, finding ways to deal with the boredom it causes should be a priority.

Why Boredom Is Different for People With ADHD

Everybody gets bored from time to time. Adults without ADHD can still find their way around tasks which they believe to be boring. Oftentimes, they do it only because they have to. For instance, they would not like to pay late fees, so they pay their bills on time. The motivation for these actions are external and they often wouldn't need an internal motivation to finish a boring task.

However, as an adult with ADHD, you cannot get through a task for which there is no internal motivation. For you, completing a task that you consider boring can only happen when you are able to identify it as boring, after which you can then work on strategies which will help you complete it.

Adults with ADHD struggle in this manner because the level of dopamine in their system is abnormally low. Simply the amount of stimulation your brain gets is not enough for it to carry out tasks. Together with the incredibly low levels of dopamine, your brain's reward center is not triggered if there is no internal interest in the activity, because there is no release of dopamine.

The lack of or low production of dopamine makes a person with ADHD easily bored. Sometimes boredom sets in because the brain records the reward as being too distant. In this case, the moment you feel that the reward is close or readily available, you will act upon it.

However, you can not project beyond your present moment due to problems with your working and long-term memory. This will make you ignore and lose sight of your long-term goals. This occurs mostly when the task that leads up to the desired goal is boring.

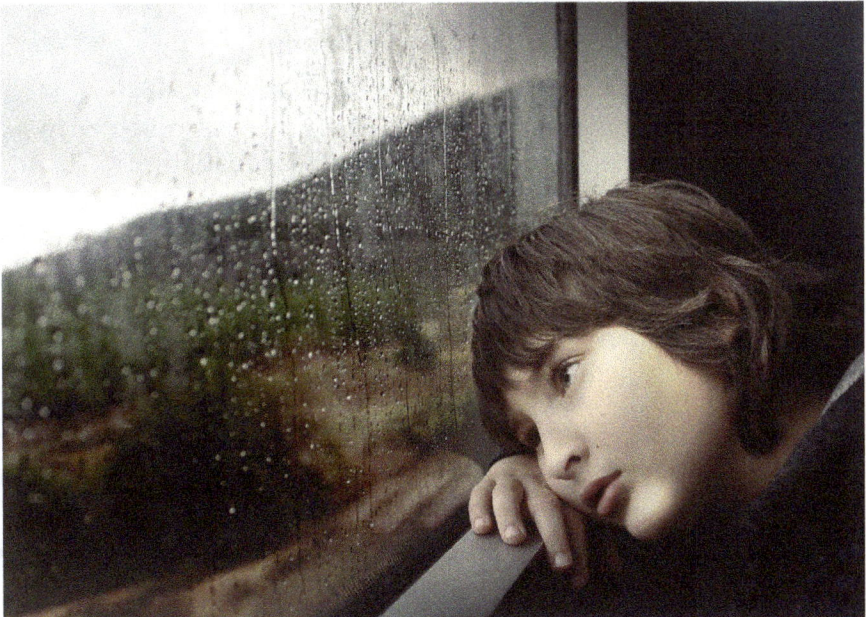

For instance, you have been assigned to work on a very important project. You are aware that this project will be helpful to you. The fact that the stimulus is presented and the reward is instant will make it easier for you to approach the task. In this case, your brain has received stimulation and the promised rewards triggers motivation. However, if you cannot form a direct connection with the reward at that point, there is no chance of completing the task.

Here's a typical ADHD attitude:

1. You pass by your bathroom on your way to your work desk. You think, The bathroom needs cleaning. I should get it done then I can return to work.
2. After cleaning the bathroom, you start preparing to work, then you get a Facebook notification and think, I should take a little break before I begin.
3. While checking the notifications, you get an email and then you decide that those need to be answered first.

In this scenario, you're getting the stimulus and reward of cleaning the bathroom, and checking your notifications and email instantly. The benefits are right at your feet. Your neglect of the long-term task is because the reward is not instant. This makes the task boring and so you have no interest in doing it.

By now, you should understand that ADHD has an influence on your feelings of boredom. But then, if everyone feels bored anyway, why do people with ADHD feel extremely incapable of tolerating boredom?

The brain with ADHD yearns for stimulation. As a person with ADHD, your brain is actively seeking different means to get the fix it needs. So, when your brain needs an excessive amount of stimulation, it places you under intense physiological stress because it is poorly stimulated.

This forces you to go in search of extra stimulation to reduce your boredom. The method you choose to satisfy your boredom should be taken into consideration. For instance, you could choose to exercise vigorously or take up a healthy hobby. On the other hand, your boredom might push you to satisfy your brain needs through risky habits like excessive eating, compulsive spending, playing video games excessively, starting an argument, providing a 'crisis' response, and many more.

If you find yourself getting involved in more risky behavior due to your brain's need for stimulation, you will need to be more intentional about your actions. You will need to learn to form habits that delegate the responsibility of choosing a stimulating activity to your intellect and not your brain wiring.

However, if your brain doesn't cooperate with your decision, it throws you into more dilemmas. This is why Dr. Ellen Littman, a clinical psychologist and ADHD expert, suggests that the treatment for ADHD should focus on learning how to make the brain conform and attend to urgent low stimulation activities. You will need some strategies to achieve that:

- **Learn to identify what your boredom feels like:** You cannot manage a situation that you know nothing about. To manage your boredom, you should learn to know when you are bored. For some people with ADHD, boredom comes as frustration. And in this case, they can point out their frustration. However, they fail to identify that their boredom is causing the frustration. For some people, this boredom-turned-frustration eventually becomes anger.

  → Some people feel tired when they are actually bored. And when they take a nap, the boredom increases. The cycle created is harmful. Boredom can also feel like excessive restlessness. You begin to feel pumped with so much energy and no idea what to do with it. If you are able to detect it at this point, you could channel it into positive activities. The key to managing your boredom is realizing what it really feels like.

- **Discover your boredom routine:** After learning to recognize how you feel when you're bored, you should figure out your boredom routine. What is the pattern of your reaction when you're bored? Think deeply if you feel you don't have a boredom routine.

Do you do any of the following:

- Check your facebook app?
- Do simple work that is not urgent?
- Focus intensely on whatever your attention lands on?
- Surf the internet or watch TV thoughtlessly?
- Consume alcohol or drugs?
- Oversleep?
- Overeat?
- Mindlessly skip through activities?

Your boredom routine is the set of activities that you fall back on when you are bored. Examine them, and if you don't want those activities to be your default, you'll need to make a change.

STOPPING BOREDOM

Yeah, you can actually stop being bored. Usually, your default response when boredom creeps into a task you're working on is to stop doing the task. However, you can choose the better option of preventing boredom, although you will need extra planning to achieve this.

Try using these principles to help you effectively deal with boredom:

- **Discover your main interest factors:** Do you have any interests? Note down the things that draw your interest and excitement. After that, figure out what all of those things have in common. For instance, if you are intensely excited by running, rock climbing, or hiking, the common factor is that they are outdoor activities that involve movement.

- **Incorporate key interest factors into your life:** Typically, your brain does not get pleasure from daily activities, and so you need to supply plenty of satisfaction and interest some other way. And because you cannot provide this naturally all the time, scheduling helps take the burden off you. If you can engage in at least one high interest activity to provide dopamine for your brain, you will find it easier to tolerate basic tasks.

- **Insert key interest factors in other sectors of your day:** Realistically, you cannot spend an entire day engaging in high interest activities. If you have figured out the key interest factors, you can insert them into your other tasks for the day. For instance, a person whose key factors are the outdoors and movement can introduce these things by walking outside when on a work call, or shifting their workstation outdoors occasionally.

TIPS TO FORESTALL BOREDOM

Even though you try to fight your boredom, you can use a different strategy, which is avoiding it. These tips can help you keep boredom out of your day:

- **Expect delays and setbacks:** Think about your day and picture the things that can potentially bore you to tears. How can you make your day interesting? You could read a book while you wait for the doctor or knit a scarf through a webinar. You could even walk through an afternoon Zoom meeting. Prepare beforehand and think of ways to make basic activities interesting.

- **Be your own playmate:** You can turn a portion of your basic tasks into games and competitions. If you don't like doing dishes, how about a small game? How fast can you do the dishes? Can you do it faster than the last time? If you cannot endure staff meetings, how about observing the behavior of others? How often does a member of staff clear their throat? Doing things like this helps you find some excitement in activities that would otherwise be boring.

- **Have more activities:** Your brain's first reaction to a boring and uninteresting task is to disengage, however that is counterproductive as it intensifies the boredom. When you notice the feeling during a task, ask yourself what extra thing you need to do. Do you have an extra project you can handle? Can you learn more skills? Find some other angle of the task that you are yet to explore and do it.

- **Create an activity menu:** Make a note of all your high interest activities. Are there other activities you could add, like things that share similar interest factors with the activities on your list, or those you have been longing to try out? Keep the activity menu available for when you're bored so you can try them out.

WHAT TO DO WHEN YOU FEEL BORED

So what if you get bored right in the middle of an important task? How do you work through it rather than abandoning the task?

Do this: Build the right environment to reduce feelings of boredom. First, you need to figure out the tasks that are boring to you. After that, you can then create a plan to help you trudge through them. Usually, you would fall back to your boredom routine and get away from the task, but the following strategies can help you out:

- Understand that everyday you do not have an infinite amount of will power and it diminishes as the day goes by. To utilize this properly, start your day doing the boring tasks before you exhaust all your willpower.

- Find an accountability partner to keep you in check as you work even on boring tasks. Be accountable to yourself by sharing your activities regularly with someone who supports you.

- Give yourself rewards often. Take a break after a long period of working rather than waiting until the end. You can take a walk to help you relax.

- Create a short timeframe to complete your task so it does not overwhelm you. Also, try to make your work a little fun if possible. Set up your workspace in a serene environment but place enough stimuli for your brain. While you try to avoid distractions, provide some stimulation for your brain.

- Time your task to be linked to the period you have to take your medication. Create a time for play so you are motivated to do your work or see it as interesting.

- Find something to occupy your drifting attention. Give your mind simple or complex tasks to accomplish which helps reduce boredom.

- Though you may try, putting all your interest in boring activities can be overwhelming, regardless of the goals you need to meet. Your attention drifts probably because your brain is searching for stimulation. And when you do not occupy that part of your brain, it may trigger you to say or do something to stimulate itself. Those things may not be appropriate for the situation. So if your brain is bored and looking for a high, occupy it with something like music or a fidgeting object.

• Think about the reward after accomplishing the goal. If a task becomes boring to you, think about what you can gain at the end. Focusing on the reward will help you continue even when you don't feel like it. When you get bored of a task, you might want to interpret that task as being less important to you.

If you consider a task to be boring and uninteresting, it does nothing to take away the importance of a project. However, your ADHD can increase your difficulty of continuing even when you're thinking about the goal. So, the best way of continuing the task is to picture your goal as being close by and readily available for you.

When the feelings of boredom arrive and you try to decide if you are to continue with it or not, you might forget your goal. Picturing the goal as almost close to reality can help you. Here are some tips to help you connect to your goal and choose it over your boredom:

• Build a graphic of images and words and place it on a visible spot.
• Include a note when you create a reminder on your calendar for the task.
• Make an electronic visual of your goal to sit on the screen of your devices.
• Write a message on an online sticky note and include it in your default browser. This way, it is the first message you see when you go online.
• Discover other ways to remind yourself how important a project is.

Get Ready for Some Discomfort

Most of the tips emphasize on making an environment that reduces your feelings of boredom. However, this cannot always be possible and you need to learn to endure a little discomfort. If you master tolerance for discomfort, you will reduce the likelihood of participating in activities that do not align with your goals and values.

It starts like this: When you recognize the onset of your boredom, you think, "I know I don't feel good, but I'll try to keep up with this for some more time."

Getting used to the discomfort is a realistic way to deal with this because you won't always have something to stimulate you at that moment. This even helps you avoid reacting on impulse and doing something that will cause you regrets later. If you can endure the discomfort for a while, it buys you time to provide a proper response to the feelings you're having.

Take a Break to Stimulate Your Brain

If you have tried all the tips above and you still struggle with your feelings, then it's time for a break. Since you are trying to manage your disorder, you should also know when you have reached your limit of self-control. At that moment, the best thing will be to take a break and decide on how to stimulate your brain. This is not encouragement to quit the work entirely, but rather some sort of recharge period. If you ignore it at this point, your impulses might take over and create an experience or action that you would eventually regret. If you are in the middle of a meeting, request that the meeting is reconvened or excuse yourself if that is not possible. If you work alone, take some time off to do some activity (other than work, of course) that you like.

ADHD AND SELF-CONTROL

An individual cannot successfully manage their actions, thoughts, and words in different scenarios without self-control. Self-control is the power you have to choose a response suitable for a scenario in a way that protects your goals and produces the best outcome over time. Your "executive function capacity" determines your level of self-control.

"Executive functions" refers to the mental process that allows an individual to deliberately ignore instinct or habits and respond wilfully.

Simply put, self-control is being completely responsible for all your actions, thoughts, and words, and operating above basic instincts. It means you have the ability to make decisions after consideration of their consequences.

To exhibit self-control, you need to pause instead of instinctively reacting to every stimulus. In addition, you should do these:

- Pull your attention inside of you.
- Carefully understand your internal and external states.
- Self-placate (when gratification is delayed or discomfort sets in).
- Moderate interruption of internal stimulus (thoughts, feelings) and external stimulus (sights and sounds).
- Connect past and present situations together, as well as the consequences of different responses.
- Study information, create and modify ideas, and plan the future.
- Make appropriate independent responses.

People with ADHD, especially the Hyperactive/Impulsive type, usually react directly to stimuli. Their poor executive function prevents them from pausing, understanding scenarios, and conducting themselves in any of the actions related to self-control as earlier described.

This causes them to act impulsively regardless of consequence, have problems delaying gratification, and struggle to manage their emotions.

How to Improve Self-Control

If you didn't know any better, you might join the bandwagon of those who believe that people with ADHD lack self-control just for the sake of it. However, ADHD symptoms compel the individual to act on impulse with little regard for consequence.

With ADHD medication, a person can boost their self-control. The medication improves the capacity of a person with ADHD to take a break and employ their executive functions in deciding the appropriate response or action for a scenario.

However, it is wrong to think that application of self-control alone always produces the best outcome. Still, individuals with ADHD need to learn how to utilize their self-control in situations to protect goal attainment. Adults with ADHD can employ these methods to improve self-control:

- Create strategies that trigger them to take a step back, as doing so helps them reduce the likelihood of making an impulsive action. Strategies they could use to pause upon reception of stimuli include deep breathing, visualising their lips closed, walking away, and trying to repeat the statement of the other person before replying. Constant meditation and mindfulness practice can help to induce a pause which gives the person a little control.

- Understand how their self-control affects them the most so they can be proactive about responding to situations. For instance, an impulsive person who often provides instant response to requests can practice saying, "Let me get back to you." If they are often triggered by someone, they can plan to stay away from them, or calm their emotions by repeating certain phrases in their mind.

- They can also set prompts and reminders to jolt them back into reality if they are easily distracted during tasks that involve writing.

- Get visual reminders that provide reminders of their goals, their motivations, and other things that are important. In most cases, they can split major tasks into several minor ones, and create an effective plan to utilize their time.

- Practice self-compassion and try to be kind to themselves.

- Tackle the need for perfection and embrace all their imperfections as humans—this way they can be more tolerant of their mistakes.

- Remind themselves when they behave in socially unacceptable ways that all relationships have cracks and they need to apologise, forgive themselves, and continue their life.

- Work with an accountability partner or ADHD coach that supports them and pushes them towards acknowledging and embracing their strengths and struggles, and seeking out methods to boost their self-control.

- Celebrate all the positives in their lives despite how small it seems.

SELF-CARE FOR A PERSON WITH ADHD

Self-care is very important and self-definitive. What do you imagine self-care to be? Does it mean something as simple as brushing your teeth twice daily? Do you think about a special event like a trip to a spa that includes yoga, a massage, and a pedicure?

For the most part, self-care involves parenting yourself and looking after your own well-being. It may sound good to have a spa day, but you're only indulging. Actual self-care involves the system of living. As someone with ADHD, you might consider creating a day planner and sticking to a routine, finally scheduling and honoring physician and therapist appointments, building an organizational system while also making time to review your actions, and more, and more.

Practising self-care involves scheduling time to attend to yourself and your needs. Regular self-care helps you manage stress and live your best life. Self-care should cater to these five different areas of life:

- physical needs
- safety and security
- love and belonging
- self-esteem, self-respect, and self-efficacy
- utilizing your talents and manifesting potential

For an adult with ADHD, building healthy self-care practices make up the behavioral management of ADHD. This is also known as "coping skills." These coping skills are the structures that support people to achieve life demands and stay in a positive mindset.

Physicians and mental health professionals who treat adults with ADHD supervise their patients to create self-care methods that they can practice as they respond to treatment. To achieve this, some physicians study the environment of the individual and jointly discuss ways to accommodate their realities to their needs.

The method of self-care you choose is unique for you, as there is no one-size-fits-all pattern. However, there are different approaches that correlate with one another and your treatment plan.

DEVELOPING SELF-CARE STRATEGIES

Non-superficial self-care for an adult involves being honest about your needs and the adverse impact of your ADHD on simple tasks.

Physical Needs

These are the basics. You need to look after your health, and stabilize your food, water, shelter, exercise, and clothing needs. This can be something like creating a meal schedule, adding a grocery shopping appointment in your daily planner, and much more. You need to attend to your physical needs and boost your overall health while you're at it.

Safety and Security Needs

This involves sorting out important major issues, which might require getting extra help from a therapist or financial expert. Achieving financial security is a good way of catering to your safety and security needs. Have you been saving up for a down payment on a house? Do you live in fear of a physical or environmental attack? Are you struggling emotionally with anxiety, depression, anger, and fear? Fixing any form of instability in this sector can be a form of security.

Love and Belonging

Building and maintaining positive relationships is a form of self-care. Study yourself and identify what kind of relationships you have around you. How strong are they? You can achieve a sense of belonging by joining support groups or groups with interests that you like. For instance, book clubs, knitting clubs, a foreign language club, or even a sports team.

Self-Esteem, Self-Respect, and Self-Efficacy

Have you been feeling low and down in the
dumps? Do you ever give yourself any credit at all? Self-care can involve focusing on your successes rather than your mistakes and failures. Find time to think about everything that is going on in your life, like your already accomplished goals,, and give yourself credit for

those. Another way to achieve self-care in this regard is considering your interests and rejecting activities that you don't like, people who are needy, or activities that you have no time for. You can also learn to ask for help when you need it. Although difficult, putting yourself first is a form of self-care that gets easier with time.

Manifesting Your Potential

Everyone desires to use their gifts. However, you may not realize that this is an incredible form of self-care. Create time in your schedule to outline your values and relate them to your daily actions. Do you think you're meeting up with those goals? Do you need to make changes in your current lifestyle to achieve fulfillment or completely leverage your skills?

Making Time for Your Needs

Now, while you need to improve on several areas of your life as a form of self-care, you also need to avoid rushing it. Go one step at a time and figure out the things that have gone right or wrong. The best way to make changes is to focus on the reward. You can't change everything at once, and rather than panicking, note all the things you can achieve in the moment.

Self-care is essential and without it you will feel depleted in different sectors of your life. Convince yourself of how valuable you are. Many people with ADHD have difficulty putting themselves first. They . They feel their value is obtained from making others a priority and only looking after themselves after they have settled others' problems.

You don't have to feel like you don't deserve self-care or there is no time for that. As a person with ADHD, self-care gives you an amount of control over an aspect that is not common in your life. Practice self-care care as frequently as you can.

CHAPTER 7

MEDITATION AND ADHD

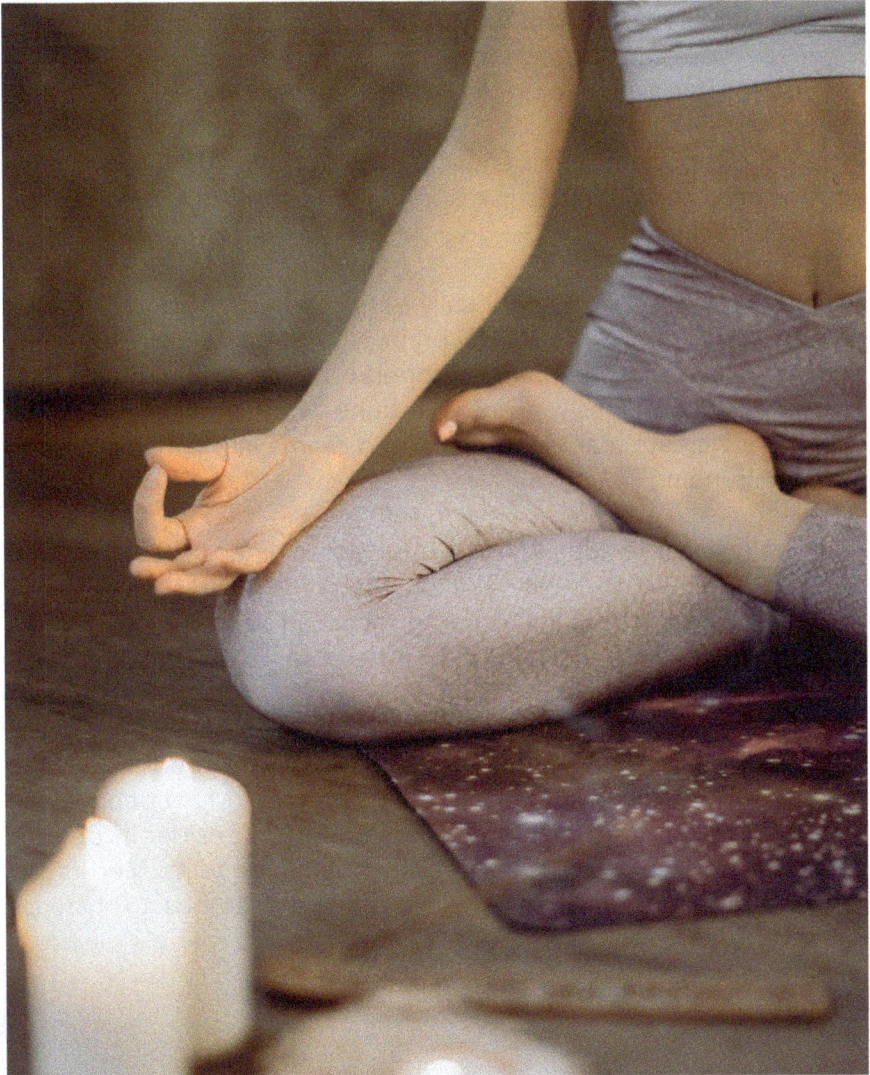

The primary treatment options offered to adults with ADHD are medication and therapy. However, they are not the only methods of combating ADHD. Meditation has been shown to provide significant improvement for people with ADHD. Meditation is a practice involving various methods with the aim of cultivating attention and awareness to reach a clear and stable emotional and mental state.

Many people with ADHD seem to be uninterested in the practice, probably because of the misconceptions about it. It's hard for them to imagine a practice where they have to do 'nothing' the entire time. However, you can practice meditation without getting into the famous lotus position or doing some uncomfortable acts. While people with ADHD may see meditation as difficult, the practice is incredibly important and beneficial. If you have ADHD, you have accumulated certain habits in response to your ADHD, which affects your general life.

Most people with ADHD habitually run on adrenaline. For the most part it starts like this: The ADHD brain is constantly sleepy. Then the person realizes that the brain is triggered to wake when it's excited. Then they unconsciously fall into a routine where they create regular crises. They create fear, excitement, and drama in their lives to keep the brain running.

Technically, people with ADHD abuse adrenaline rushes and soon become addicted to them. The process of awakening the sleepy frontal lobes with stress and other triggers can be detrimental to the body. It affects the heart rate, blood pressure, blood sugar, and the immune system in general.

While this ADHD activity can be managed with medication and therapy, meditation can be incredibly helpful too. Many people with ADHD find relief from practicing meditation.. CConsider it. Besides relief from ADHD, you will also get other health benefits. Medication can be combined with your main treatment methods to increase effectiveness.

MYTHS ABOUT MEDITATION

There are several misconceptions about the practice of meditation. However, if you intend to practice meditation, you need to have correct information. These are some of the debunked myths surrounding meditation.

There Is Only One Kind of Meditation

No. There are several kinds of meditation, and you can practice any kind that is suitable for you. This myth is probably fueled by the idea that people just sit and close their eyes during meditation. However, only a few kinds of meditation involve the widely known 'lotus' position. Some meditation involves slow and gentle movements.

Others focus on visualization and mantras. Some meditation is incorporated into daily activities. There are many different kinds of meditation for you to embrace.

Meditation Will Provide Instant Relief

Even though meditation is effective, the process is gradual. It is not a smooth journey to achieve a still mind. When you start the process and progress to an advanced level, you gain knowledge of unhealthy mental habits. This awareness can trigger some unpleasant effects like anxiety or disorientation. The experience can however be managed by practicing under a qualified meditation guide. The most important thing to note though is that meditation is not going to provide instant results.

Meditation Must Be Practiced in Silence

For most people, meditation means sitting still and breathing in silence. However, this is just one kind of meditation. There are several other forms of meditation which involve various degrees of movement. In meditation, you are trying to quell your thoughts and concentrate on your breath. Although you want to have a quiet and calm mind, your body doesn't have to be still or quiet.

Meditation Is Practiced Just to Clear the Mind

In meditation, you're studying your mind and trying to gain better control of it through awareness of thought. After a thorough awareness, you can achieve mindfulness. The different meditation practices help you detect the thought patterns which your mind creates while they are still in formation, and return peaceful concentration and awareness to the central point.

Meditation Is Relaxing

Meditation is not entirely relaxing. At first you may not feel calm or better. Sometimes, especially on the first trial, you might develop anxiety due to the discomfort of confronting your inner self. With meditation, you might realize some startling unpleasant truths about yourself. While you may feel relaxed sometimes, it helps to admit that your mind might be all over the place on some days.

Meditation Doesn't Work If Your Mind Wanders

The truth is, if you could figure out your thoughts during meditation, you had a successful practice. Meditation provides the ability to detect different parts of our internal experience and not change it. More frequent practice keeps you from being caught up in your thoughts. It helps you stay in control and at peace, but the thoughts do not fade into thin air. Most guides believe that not having thoughts during meditation means you did not notice them.

Meditation Is Hard

Although sitting and meditating for a while might seem tedious, we already meditate a lot. Meditation involves focusing the mind on a certain thing for a long time. When we watch movies or use social media, we are already doing that. But the practice involves concentrating on something that will improve our lives. It isn't as hard as you imagine.

Meditation Is Selfish

Meditation is just like sleeping and physical exercise, and therefore can only be selfish if those are. Meditation helps you exercise your mind and awareness to keep you grounded, calmer, and less reactive. The people around also benefit from your new state of mind and you become better at your work.

Meditation Makes You Weak

This thought is prominent among men who think meditation will make them less edgy and more soft. With meditation, you don't feel the flight-or-fight response and you are fully engaged in the present. This time you respond rather than react. With meditation, your focus and performance is improved. Even sports players practise meditation, therefore there is nothing to worry about and it does not make you weak and it does not make you weak.

Meditation Must Be Done Sitting

You can do meditation anytime. Moving, sitting, standing, it's all up to you and the kind of meditation practise you choose. The benefits of practising meditation when you're moving is the same as doing it when sitting, and even comes with the added benefit of improving digestion, circulation, and blood flow.

You Suck at Meditation

There are many forms of meditation and no single right or wrong way to do it. Meditation practice is named so because you're practicing the skills of monitoring and focusing attention. You can't exactly be bad or good at it. The goal is to help you learn new ways to respond to your thoughts, and help your brain master new thoughts and patterns—not to stop your thoughts altogether.

Meditation Is a Religious Activity

Meditation has its roots in religion. Many religions embrace it, too. Still, it can be practiced outside religion. Some people regard meditation as a spiritual act without adding the dogma or rules of religion. Therefore, you can practise meditation regardless of your religious beliefs.

Meditation Takes Hours

No, you don't have to spend several hours practicing meditation or hide yourself away somewhere. You can practice meditation for five minutes or as long as it is comfortable for you.

TYPES OF MEDITATION

As has been mentioned earlier, you don't have to restrict yourself to one kind of meditation. These are the various kinds of meditation you can engage in.

Spiritual Meditation

Meditation is integral in Eastern spiritual traditions. However, it is also recognized in several Judeo-Christian traditions. Some forms of spoken, silent, or chanted prayer can be regarded as spiritual meditation. Meditation fosters a deeper connection with the divine if practised in a religious setting. Buddhism and Taoism are non-theistic ways of life and they practice meditation for self-awareness.

People who practise non-theistic spiritual meditation learn to become the best versions of themselves. Spiritual meditation teaches you benevolence and connection. It can be practiced at home, in nature, or at a place of worship. If you desire self-reflection and spiritual growth, then you can practice different forms of spiritual meditation.

Mindfulness Meditation

Mindfulness meditation is now a widespread practice in the West and has its roots in the teachings of the Buddha. Mindfulness meditation helps us learn how the mind operates. The knowledge we gain from the practice can improve the quality of our lives by helping us embrace patience, tolerance, and many other positive values. To perfect mindfulness, you need to learn to acknowledge your present, observe and recognize your thoughts, focus on your object of meditation, and appreciate the moment you are in. Mindfulness meditation also involves concentration and awareness.

You need to get into a disciplined meditation posture (usually the lotus position) with a straight back,, and embrace the desire to be true to yourself. Your breath is the best focus for mindfulness meditation. If you find your thoughts drifting, return them to your breath without judgment.

Movement Meditation

Movement meditation is practiced during motion. Unlike other forms of meditation where you need to be in one position, the focus for this type of meditation is the moving body. This meditation technique is used in yoga, tai chi, other martial arts, and other martial arts, and walking.. You need to be fully present in your body as you practice. Your awareness can be extended to other activities where you are in motion, like gardening, playing games, walking your dog, etc. The most important thing is that you make your moving body the object. Focus on your practice.

Focused Meditation

This kind of meditation encourages you to focus exclusively on your present activity. Simply put, you're monotasking instead of multitasking. It is a common belief that multitasking helps us feel like superhumans who can handle a lot of things at once. However, during multitasking, our thoughts are all over the place and we are often dissatisfied.

One commonly practiced type of focus meditation is drinking a cup of tea. To do this, you train yourself to ignore all other activities and concentrate completely on the cup of tea in your hands. If your mind drifts, you guide it lovingly back to the tea drinking.

This practice is not limited to drinking tea. You can do this when you are eating, working out, or doing other activities. Committing to this practice will improve your ability to concentrate.

Visualization Meditation

This meditation technique involves concentrating the mind on a certain quality or feeling. On a basic level, you just have to close your eyes and think of something pleasant. Your mind can create an image of something calming and relatable. It could be a garden of flowers, a beautiful mountain lake or the open sky, your favorite location, or any other visualization that works for you.

During this exercise, we picture our emotions and thoughts as leaves on a stream being swept downstream in the most gentlest of ways. This visualization helps protect you from distracting mental activity. Formally, visualization meditation is a specific religious practice in the Tibetan tradition. It is a complex spiritual practice which requires the guidance of a skilled teacher.

The visualization meditation uses the mind's creative power to cause positive personal change.

Chanting Meditation

Different religions and spiritualities encourage chanting and mantra meditation. In this case, the mind concentrates on the sound of the words and melody. Different traditions have specific focus when using mantras. You can use a mantra accompanied by a melody or one without. The most common sound in mantra meditation is 'Om.' People who enjoy chanting meditation mantras develop an alert mind that is still calm and peaceful. The spirituality aspect of chanting meditation helps strengthen your connection to positive human values and you will need a teacher to guide you.

BENEFITS OF MEDITATION FOR PEOPLE WITH ADHD

Just like muscles, the brain can be made stronger with exercise. With meditation, you can learn to control your attention and redirect your mind to the present. This improves your emotional awareness and reduces your chances of acting impulsively.

For ADHD in particular, meditation thickens the prefrontal cortex which is responsible for focus, impulse control, and planning. It increases the brain's level of dopamine which the brain with ADHD has small amounts of. According to research, mindfulness meditation can reduce major ADHD symptoms. In a recent study, people with ADHD who practice home meditation noticed an increase in their concentration. They had less depression and anxiety symptoms, too. Besides specific ADHD benefits, meditation supports weight loss, stress reduction, and an increased self-esteem.

People with ADHD often have trouble remembering stuff and this increases self-criticism. However, meditation helps them become less self-judgemental. It reduces the amount of stress hormones that are produced during situations that typically have resulted in anxiety. Mindfulness meditation can allow you to lose some weight because now you're more aware and careful about the things you eat.

WHY MEDITATION CAN BE HARD FOR PEOPLE WITH ADHD

ADHD symptoms make meditation more difficult. It is harder for people with ADHD to keep their focus stable. These are some of the disturbances they may experience during meditation:

- a heightened awareness of symptoms followed by anxiety
- introspection that may give rise to negative self-talk
- feelings of being overwhelmed
- boredom
- restlessness/fidgeting
- trouble ignoring the symptoms of others in group sessions

Generally, ADHD makes the individual feel like two minutes is a long time. And in the event where there is no immediate relief or effects, the individual feels frustrated and may quit the practice before the point where it becomes beneficial. However, working with a good meditation guide will help you overcome your obstacles during the practice.

HOW TO MEDITATE EFFECTIVELY

Even if you have a restless brain, you can still reap the benefits of meditation using the following steps.

Encourage Yourself

Reaffirm your readiness to practice meditation. Repeat to yourself as many times as you like: "Meditation is a practice. I will enjoy and reap the benefits of the experience. I refuse to judge myself because there is no wrong way to do it."

Be Comfortable

You probably have heard that you don't need to be too comfortable so you don't fall asleep. However, if you sleep during the practice, you probably need it. Set an alarm if you're worried you'll sleep off and miss something important.

Create Your Comfort Zone

Depending on the type of meditation practice, you should choose positions that are comfortable for you. You don't need to be distracted by physical discomfort.

Breathe Slowly and Evenly

In the beginning, your breath may feel rushed and uneven. The more relaxed you become, the slower it gets.

Get Off the Adrenaline Mode

Don't meditate if you are already worked up. Find a way to settle down first. You might take a hot bath or listen to soothing music. While you settle down, get into comfortable clothing and remove accessories that might make you uncomfortable.

Change Your Mental State Using Sensory Cues

You might use some kinds of music, a special hat, chair, or something else to help you ease into meditation.

Select Your Focus Object

You will need to channel your focus somewhere while you meditate. This could be your breathing, or a phrase or visual cue. People with ADHD have difficulty using visual focus. However, it may be different for you. Choose what you are most comfortable with.

Music Can be Your Focus Too

Meditation focus can be musical. A good recommendation is Steven Halpern's music. Use only instrumentals so you don't become distracted by lyrics.

Moving Meditation or Sitting Meditation—Your Choice

Forget the stereotype for meditation and go for the most suitable option for you. People with ADHD do better with moving meditation to prevent distraction from your restless body. It will be great if you use a simple, repetitive movement like walking.

Get Into the Meditation Mood

Even if you're prepared to meditate, your thoughts may fight for your attention. If that happens, gently disengage your attention from the distraction and return your focus. You may experience this a lot in the beginning or on bad brain days.

Maintain Your Practice

The more you practice, the easier it gets. You just have to proceed gradually. You can start with five minutes a few times daily. If you get comfortable, you can increase your practice duration.

Complete relaxation is easily achieved after you have fully entered meditation mode. You might achieve this with a few deep breaths and this will help you in situations where you feel overwhelmed.

Remind Yourself the Reason for Your Practice

You are meditating to move out of the noise and concentrate on a focus object, not to clear your mind.

Take Your Medication First

With a suitable dose of a stimulant medicine, you can reduce brain activity and help yourself get ready for meditation.

Make It a Routine

Making meditation a routine is a great idea. However, if you have problems following a routine, work with a coach. A meditation coach guides your practice and keeps you on track.

Get Off Your Phone

Ensure that you are practicing in a quiet spot without distractions. Make sure you are not bothered by alerts and notifications from your electronic devices. You can go into an empty space just to be alone for your practice.

Work With the Environment You Have

While it is recommended to use a quiet place, you may live in a busy area making that hard to achieve. Regardless, you can still meditate by shutting out the noise and concentrating on your breathing patterns. It may help to use soft music or a guided meditation app.

Observe Your Breathing

You can maintain your presence in the present moment through your breathing.mFirst, exhale and inhale naturally. Observe how your body feels. Then breathe in deeply, and again observe how your body feels. Did you notice your tummy swell? How about the fullness of your chest? Hold your breath for some seconds, then breathe out gently until you're done. Observe how your body feels with the exhale. Remember that it's okay for your mind to wander during practice as long as you return your focus to your breath.

Close Your Practice Slowly

No matter how long your practice was, take some extra time to return to the present. Allow some time to pick up what's going on around you. Also, observe how your body feels. Finally, acknowledge your emotions and thoughts.

~ CONCLUSION ~

Now that you have finished this book, you must surely have more information about ADHD than you started with. Hopefully, you have learned how ADHD manifests, the symptoms, and the diagnosis. All the information in this book was compiled from research and experience of the author. However, it's important to remember that the studies on ADHD in adults are not yet as numerous as in children. The condition in general still has a lot to be understood as there is no noted cause.

Again, there are still uncertainties regarding the exact relationship between childhood and adult ADHD. More understanding is also needed in the area of treatment. In all, research into ADHD is continuous and there's still a lot to learn. However, this book has compiled much of what is known about this disorder to help you understand and manage it. So far from this book, you have learned that

1. ADHD is a neurodevelopmental disorder which begins in childhood and sometimes continues to manifest in adulthood. It is characterized by inattention, impulsivity, and hyperactivity among other symptoms. These major symptoms also form the three types of ADHD. ADHD in adults can coexist with different psychological conditions which increases the severity.

2. ADHD should be diagnosed by a qualified mental health professional based on DSM-5 and other diagnostic criteria. There are some risk factors for ADHD, but the disorder is believed to be a combination of genetic and environmental triggers.

3. The ADHD brain is wired differently from that of a person without ADHD, hence should not be attributed to behavioral inadequacies. The treatment and management of ADHD differs based on individual needs, but medication is usually the first line of action. Most people combine medications with behavioral therapy and other methods. Eventually, with constant support and management, people with ADHD can improve the quality of their life.

Attention Deficit Hyperactive Disorder is quite treatable and people with the disorder should not be stigmatized. Hopefully, reading this book has helped you learn how to manage your ADHD or support your loved ones who live with the condition.

ACTION STEP

—

DAILY PRODUCTIVITY PLANNER

Scan the QR code or use the link to download your
daily productivity planner to track your goals, accomplishments
and schedule.

https://bit.ly/301XMcB

~REFERENCES~

All images sourced from [Pixabay, Unsplash, Pexels, Shutterstock].

Bhargava, D. H. (2021, March 10). *Attention Deficit Hyperactivity Disorder: Causes of ADHD.* WebMD. https://www.webmd.com/add-adhd/adhd-causes

Causes of ADHD: What We Know Today. (2019, September 27). American Academy of Pediatrics. https://www.healthychildren.org/English/health-issues/conditions/adhd/Pages/Causes-of-ADHD.aspx

Collingwood, J. (2016, May 17). *The Genetics of ADHD.* Psych Central. https://psychcentral.com/lib/the-genetics-of-adhd#1

Godman, H. (2014, April 9). *Regular Exercise Changes the Brain to Improve Memory, Thinking Skills.* Harvard Health Publishing. https://www.health.harvard.edu/blog/regular-exercise-changes-brain-improve-memory-thinking-skills-201404097110

Grow Out of ADHD? Not Likely. (2020, December 17). CHADD. https://chadd.org/adhd-weekly/grow-out-of-adhd-not-likely/

Holland, K. (2018, July 28). *ADHD by the Numbers: Facts, Statistics, and You.* Healthline. https://www.healthline.com/health/adhd/facts-statistics-infographic

Issa, M. T. (2021, November 23). *Adults With ADHD at Higher Risk of Developing Generalized Anxiety Disorder: Study.* Alarabiya News. https://english.alarabiya.net/News/world/2021/11/23/Adults-with-ADHD-at-higher-risk-of-developing-generalized-anxiety-disorder-Study

Love, T. (2020, April). *Internet Addiction and ADHD.* CHADD. https://chadd.org/adhd-news/adhd-news-adults/internet-addiction-and-adhd/

Stieg, G. (2019, September 15). *Fitness Literally Boosts Your Brainpower, According to a New Study.* CNBC. https://www.cnbc.com/2019/09/15/exercise-benefits-cognitive-function-performance.html

Sublet, A. (2020, October 27). *The Healing Power of Singing.* The New York Times. https://www.nytimes.com/2020/10/27/well/mind/choir-singing-music-anxiety-stress.html

Weinstock, P. C. (2017, December 29). Cigarette Smoking During Pregnancy Linked to ADHD Risk in Offspring. Reuters. https://www.reuters.com/article/us-health-pregnancy-smoking-adhd-idUSKBN1EN1M9